THE DIABETES CURE
2-IN-1 BUNDLE

Diabetes Diet Solution + Weight Loss Affirmations- The #1 Complete Box Set to Control Your Blood Sugar, Cease Bad Habits, and Stay Healthy

Diabetes Diet Solution: Prevent and Reverse Diabetes

Discover How to Control Your Blood Sugar and Live Heathy, Even if You're Diagnosed with Type 1 or 2 Diabetes

By Cheryl Field

© Copyright 2018 - All rights reserved.

The following eBook is reproduced below with the goal of providing information that is as accurate and reliable as possible. Regardless, purchasing this eBook can be seen as consent to the fact that both the publisher and the author of this book are in no way experts on the topics discussed within and that any recommendations or suggestions that are made herein are for entertainment purposes only. Professionals should be consulted as needed prior to undertaking any of the action endorsed herein.

This declaration is deemed fair and valid by both the American Bar Association and the Committee of Publishers Association and is legally binding throughout the United States.

Furthermore, the transmission, duplication, or reproduction of any of the following work including specific information will be considered an illegal act irrespective of if it is done electronically or in print. This extends to creating a secondary or tertiary copy of the work or a recorded copy and is only allowed with the express written consent from the Publisher. All additional right reserved.

The information in the following pages is broadly considered a truthful and accurate account of facts and as such, any inattention, use, or misuse of the information in question by the reader will render any resulting actions solely under their purview. There are no scenarios in which the publisher or the original author of this work can be in any fashion deemed liable for any hardship or damages that may befall them after undertaking information described herein.

Additionally, the information in the following pages is intended only for informational purposes and should thus be thought of as universal. As befitting its nature, it is presented without assurance regarding its prolonged validity or interim quality. Trademarks that are mentioned are done without written consent and can in no way be considered an endorsement from the trademark holder.

Table of Contents

Introduction 6

Chapter 1: Quick Introduction to Diabetes 8

Chapter 2: Diabetic Diet: The Low-Carb Diet 27

Chapter 3: The Diabetic Food List 49

Chapter 4: Effective Low Carb Diet with Healthy Habits 73

Chapter 5: Check on Your Progression 86

Conclusion 92

Introduction

Congratulations on purchasing Diabetes Diet Solution: Prevent and Reverse Diabetes and thank you for doing so.

My intention in making this book is to impart knowledge on how diabetes can be effectively managed without reaching for medications. Type 2 diabetes can be managed through diet alone, and that is by using a diet that is low in carbs with virtually no sugar and refined carbohydrates. These foods are the main culprits of perpetuating the disease in our society. If you eat these foods regularly, I urge you to stop because you are doing more harm than you may realize.

In chapter one, I give a general yet comprehensive overview of what diabetes is, its origins, and its main mechanisms. Though I used medical terms and other specialized vocabularies, I will assume that you have no biology training. I will try to explain concepts in the simplest terms I can manage.

Chapter two will introduce you to the low-carb diet. You will learn a few different diets that are low-carb, high fat, and moderate protein. These diets have been proven to lower weight and control diabetes. My aim is to convince you to at least give some of these diets a try. If you are familiar with dieting, you are probably familiar with losing some weight at first and then regaining it back. I promise you that the low-carb diet is not some fad. It is effective and proven.

Chapter three will go over a brief list of diabetic foods, what you should avoid and what you should incorporate into your diets. I don't go in-depth into one specific food and group of foods together by their common characteristics. If you are looking for a boring list of foods and figures, you won't find it here. Instead, I will give you actionable guidelines for choosing what foods are best for your diabetes.

Chapter four will impart the other half of the battle when it comes to diabetes. This includes the importance of exercise and a little secret weapon called fasting. You will learn about portion control and the four absolute "don'ts" for diabetes treatment.

Chapter five sort of wraps things together by encouraging you to track your progress as you go forward with your dieting and exercise routines.

Thanks again for your interest in this book. I have compiled information that I researched myself on the diabetes diet. I implore you to do your own research as well. Treatment should be a discourse, not a one-sided onslaught of information.

Every effort was made to ensure it is full of as much useful information as possible. Please enjoy!

Chapter 1: Quick Introduction to Diabetes

Diabetes is an illness that is commonly talked about but is often misunderstood. You hear people say something about their blood sugar levels going down and needing a candy or sugary drink to get them back up. This is because diabetes medication can cause blood sugar to plummet which then needs to be replenished. Other times, you hear that diabetes is caused by high blood sugar. Eating sweets and sugary pastries are said to cause diabetes. Though these foods exacerbate the condition, many health professionals will tell you that they simply cannot and do not cause diabetes. Other health professionals will tell you that these foods directly cause obesity and diabetes and that they stem from the same root causes. The problem with talking about the illness is that it is so complex that few people take the time to truly understand it. But even a layperson with little biology or medical training can understand diabetes if they begin from scratch.

This chapter will give a brief overview of the disease, its origins, and how it is generally treated. Whether you are somebody who has it, or somebody you know suffers from it, you can rest assured that a greater understanding will help you deal with it. The good news is that diabetes is completely manageable given proper treatment and lifestyle choices that you will learn throughout the rest of the book.

Conventional wisdom says that diabetes is caused by eating sugary foods. After all, diabetics suffer from high blood sugar, so it makes sense. Taking this further, it is easy to say that diabetes is a modern illness. Go to any gas station or corner store and have a look around the food they sell there. Candy, sugary sports and energy drinks, pastries, Cinnabons, etc. You name it. Go to any grocery store and what do you see? Aisles of refined carbs like pasta, bread, baked goods and a plethora of other "healthy" cheeses, meats, and snacks that are highly processed. Breakfast cereals are loaded with sugars and high-fructose corn syrup. Our modern lives are saturated with so much sugar that it is no mystery why diabetes is everywhere.

Despite the modern undertones, few realize that diabetes is an ancient disease. The earliest depiction of diabetes comes from ancient Egypt in a manuscript where it is described by its most recognizable symptom: excessive urination. The Greek physician Apollonius of Memphis would later give the disease a name. Diabetes literally means to "pass through" or "siphon" in Ancient Greek. No doubt this is a reference to the constant urination patients suffer from as the kidneys try to rid excess blood sugar through urine. Then in 1675, physician Thomas Willis added the term "mellitus" meaning "honey" or "sweetened with honey" in Latin. In those days, the principal way of diagnosing diabetes was through tasting the patient's urine which had a sweet taste. Diabetes Mellitus is the correct medical term used today for a group of metabolic disorders that share some characteristics but are also classified as different conditions. These incarnations of the disease only serve to complicate things further.

Some clues behind the nature of the disease are distilled in these ancient accounts. While in the Egyptian Ebbers papyrus, cancer is marked with no cure, diabetes is prescribed with a concoction of milk, berries, and plant fibers. The ancients understood that diabetes had something to do with food consumption, but the full details wouldn't be fleshed out until centuries later. In the meantime, ancient concoctions probably did very little to manage blood sugar levels. That the urine was sweet probably gave away the clue that the patient ate too much sweetened food. It could also mean that there was some internal dysfunction that caused sugar to be at high levels in the body. Regardless, it was clear that ancient physicians believed diabetes to be curable. The presence of malignant tumors meant certain death, but diabetes was more lenient a prognosis.

Unfortunately, as with cancer, there was no adequate form of treatment for diabetes back then. Patients slowly lost weight until they eventually perished. One Greek physician went on to say that diabetes was "a melting down of flesh and limbs into urine". Harrowing, but it doesn't say anything about how the disease could be cured. There is a long history of treatments that were developed from ancient times to early industrial society. Some saw limited successes, while others were downright catastrophic failures. Not surprisingly, these treatments often had to do with diet. A Scottish military surgeon prescribed all meat, low carb diets to diabetes and saw some results. Another more unfortunate French physician prescribed sugar because he thought diabetes was the excessive loss of it through urination. Of course, prescribing more sugar to a diabetic only makes their symptoms worse and accelerates the disease.

Prescribing sugar to these patients was completely unethical, but how could a 19th-century physician have known any better? The symptoms of diabetes were well-established by this time. And from those symptoms, various physicians formulated their idea of what could be causing the disease. After centuries of experimentation and progress in medical science, our picture of diabetes is much clearer now than what it was in the past. There are known treatments to help deal with the symptoms and even cure the disease altogether. While diabetes is a chronic disease, most physicians will tell you that it is incurable. Others will say that diabetic conditions are reversible, and perhaps, that alone is a form of a cure. But to understand why or why not diabetes may be cured or reversed, we need to do a deeper analysis of the disease.

Diabetes is essentially the presence of high blood sugar in the body. Blood sugar or "glucose" is the main energy source in mammals. You can think about it in terms of food for cells. Another good metaphor is gasoline and the individual cells are tanks. Without enough glucose, the body cannot perform all of its daily tasks like regulating temperature, creating new cells, and organ function. If you have too much glucose, however, the body suffers from glucotoxicity. After all, too much of a good thing results in a bad thing. Since glucose travels through the blood, glucotoxicity affects literally every part of the body. Diabetics suffer from a myriad of glucotoxicity related disorders, which are related to the size of blood vessels.

Small blood vessel or microvascular complications include retinopathy, or "diabetics eye" where the small blood vessels behind the retina become damaged. The damaged blood vessels leak blood and other fluids and eventually scar. It is the buildup of these scar tissues that cause the retina to slightly move out of place and can lead to full on blindness. Neuropathy or diabetic kidney disease occurs when the kidney can no longer clean the toxins in the blood. When these toxins are allowed to build up, they result in weight loss, nausea, and vomiting. Kidney disease is fatal if not treated. It also directly leads to end-stage renal disease, a condition characterized by the kidneys losing more than 90% of their function. A dialysis machine is needed to clean the toxins from the blood multiple times a week. Unfortunately, once the kidneys have gone this route, they will not recover unless the patient receives a transplant.

Diabetic nerve damage or neuropathy is far more common in patients. It occurs when excess blood glucose levels damage the nerve cells. The results are tingling, numbness, burning, and pain felt in the extremities and other parts of the body. In severe cases, neuropathy can be debilitating. Even powerful narcotic painkillers do little to treat these symptoms in the most severe form. Like with kidney damage, damage to the nerves cannot be repaired or reversed. The only effective treatment is to prevent the damage in the first place. This is why knowing your blood sugar levels are so important.

Large blood vessel or macrovascular complications include the hardening of arteries, a condition called atherosclerosis. This happens when the arteries are backed up by fatty material that then hardens inside the blood vessel walls. As you can imagine, this condition directly leads to heart disease, stroke, and heart attack. It should be noted that this hardening is not due to cholesterol. Instead, it results from the body's response to fix the blood vessels damaged by excess blood glucose. There is an inflammatory response to repair the damage that involves the secretion of the protein collagen and creation of smooth muscle. Cholesterol is also secreted, but it is not the prime cause of the hardening. Risk factors include smoking, high blood pressure, and of course, diabetes.

Probably the most notable complication and indeed most feared is the heart attack. Hardened arteries block off the normal flow of blood that the heart pumps. When oxygen cannot get to the vital smooth muscle cells of the heart, then they begin to die. While heart disease fatalities have been going down in the normal population, fatalities are up for diabetics.

Similarly, a stroke happens when blood vessels in the brain cannot supply oxygen anymore. Depending on the conditions of the stroke suffered, they can be disabling. Damage done to the brain cannot be repaired after large portions have died from oxygen starvation.

Another condition related to the hardening of blood vessels is called peripheral vascular disease, and it deals primarily with the disrupted blood flow to the legs by the large arteries. This condition is particularly debilitating because the patient slowly loses functions of their legs. Performing exercise becomes harder until it is impossible to do any physical activity whatsoever. In the worse cases, limbs have to be amputated to stave off infection. If there is a poor blood supply to the feet, damaged skin becomes harder to heal. Diabetic patients need to take extra care of their feet because even small cuts can develop into ulcers. Since the blood supply is disrupted, the body cannot repair itself like it normally can. Untreated ulcers may contract gangrene and need to be amputated.
As you can see, there is a myriad of complications that stem from high levels of glucose in the body. I only covered the most commonly cited ones, but rest assured that there are many more. Diabetes is characterized by an excess of glucose in the body or hyperglycemia. All of the complications and the various symptoms from the disease can be reduced to this singular mechanism. There is simply too much sugar in the blood.

Before I discuss how hyperglycemia and diabetes develops, I will differentiate between the different types of the disease. Most people have already heard about type 1 and type 2 diabetes. Those are the most common types, but others exist as well. Though different, all types of the disease have high blood sugar in common. Gestational diabetes occurs in pregnant women, caused by the excess of hormones from the placenta. There is also monogenic diabetes that is caused by a singular genetic mutation. Yet, another type of diabetes called brittle diabetes is characterized by episodes of severe low blood sugar and severe high blood sugar. For the remainder of this book, I will focus on type 1 and type 2 diabetes. Since it is more common, type 2 diabetes will be given extra attention throughout. Unless otherwise specified, the word "diabetes" as it appears in this book will refer to type 2.

The main difference between type 1 and type 2 diabetes is that type 1 is considered insulin-sensitive and type 2 diabetes is not. Insulin is a type of hormone secreted by the pancreas. It is used to tell cell receptors to allow glucose through the cell wall. Type 1 diabetes is considered an autoimmune disorder because the body's immune system has decided to attack the insulin-producing cells in the pancreas called the beta cells. Once damaged, these cells can no longer produce the insulin that is necessary to pack glucose into cells. With type 1 diabetics, insulin treatments serve to move available glucose into cells. Those who suffer from type 1 diabetes tend to lose weight more than those who have type 2. This occurs because there are low levels of insulin in the body, which forces the body to burn off fat and muscle stores at an accelerated pace because glucose isn't being used. Even if there is high glucose in the blood, it is useless without the beta cells producing the insulin required to get it into the cells.

In contrast, type 2 diabetes is considered insulin resistant. That is, the body can still freely produce insulin but has developed a tolerance against it. Blood glucose struggles to get into cells because, for whatever reason, they have developed a resistance to it. In both diseases, the primary goal of treatment is to lower the overall blood glucose level. The most effective way to do this is to prescribe insulin treatments. In the case of type 1, the role of insulin is obvious. The body is deprived of it, so an artificial source needs to be administered. In type 2 diabetes, the role of insulin is a little bit more nuanced. Insulin is already high in type 2 diabetics because the pancreas needs to work overtime to get past the insulin resistant cells. Adding more insulin into that system allows insulin resistance to be temporarily overcome.

Type 1 diabetes is believed to be caused by genetic factors, but little is understood about the mechanisms. This explains why it has a high prevalence in children and is often called juvenile diabetes. We aren't really sure what causes the body to form the autoimmune response against beta cells yet, but there are many different theories. In the US, only 5% of all diabetes diagnoses are attributed to type 1 while the vast majority (about 95%) is attributed to type 2 diabetes. What's more, up to fifty percent of the US population either suffers from diabetes or has pre-diabetic conditions that with time will develop into full-blown diabetes. In other words, America is suffering from what has been called a "diabetes epidemic" since the 1970s. The trend has spilled into other parts of the world and it is now a global phenomenon. But if only 5% of all diabetes cases are type 1 which are due to genetics, what is the cause of the other 95%?

Type 2 diabetes may also have some genetic factors involved, but it is closely associated with lifestyle choices. People aren't just born with excessive levels of glucose in their system. Neither has diabetes been so prevalent in the entire history of the world. These two factors serve as vital clues for figuring out why and how type 2 diabetes develops. First, glucose needs to somehow enter the body. This directly correlates with diet and the type of foods you choose to eat. Second, there have to be some necessary conditions present in the world for type 2 diabetes to be on the rise. The simple answer is sugar and refined carbohydrates have invaded the human diet. Sugar has always existed throughout history, but only in modern times has it been used in virtually every type or processed food. Also, I would argue that only in recent times, people have been programmed to crave it all the time. The same can be said for refined carbohydrates which are produced by mechanical and industrial processes that have only been around starting in the 19th and 20th century.

Let me break down what happens when you consume sugar and refined carbohydrates. Glucose is used as food by cells. Glucose is a type of simple sugar or monosaccharide. In contrast, the stuff you eat in food or table sugar is sucrose. Sucrose is a disaccharide or a mixture of two different sugars. It is made up of one glucose molecule and one fructose. Glucose can be directly used up as energy, but fructose cannot. Fructose needs to first be converted into glucose by the liver. You have probably heard about fructose before. It is the same sugar found in fruits. The reason why sugar is particularly bad for you is that the liver needs to work hard to convert fructose into usable energy. The more sugar you consume, the more overloaded the liver becomes. Glucose is metabolized quickly and transported in the blood to organs, muscles, and brains. Essentially, glucose is transported anywhere that needs energy. However, when there is too much glucose with not enough energetic needs, the liver stores it into glycogen. So now the liver is storing glycogen and it is still dealing with the fructose. At some point, these excess sugars cannot be used up before the next onslaught of calories is consumed. The liver then converts fructose and glycogen into fat.

Sugar is a type of carbohydrate. A carbohydrate is basically just a chain of different sugars linked up together. These sugars that make up carbohydrates cause glucose levels to spike. This is especially true for refined or "pure" carbohydrates that have been stripped off of trace amounts of the other macronutrients, those being proteins and fats. Additionally, the refining process strips any fiber present in the grain, the indigestible plant matter that makes food slower to digest. This purity of carbohydrate causes refined carbs to digest incredibly fast.

Eating either sugary or highly refined foods causes your blood glucose to spike. This, in turn, causes the pancreas to secrete insulin to diffuse that glucose into cells. Remember what I said earlier about glucotoxicity. The body realizes that high levels of glucose need to be brought down, so the right amount of insulin is released. The problem with this is that the body becomes used to the amount of insulin secreted and will require greater amounts of the hormone to metabolize glucose. Doubtless, you have heard about antibiotics resistance. The same principles apply to insulin resistance. It is essentially caused by exposure. The more antibiotics a bacterium is exposed to, the less of an effect the antibiotics have. If you regularly eat sugary and or highly refined carbs, you will develop insulin resistance over time, period. But this resistance takes years to develop. In fact, for insulin resistance to develop, a person must first suffer from hyperinsulinemia, or high levels of insulin relative to glucose in the blood.

Hyperinsulinemia is a common condition during the prediabetes stage. It is also a symptom of other metabolic diseases, the most notable being diabetes and metabolic syndrome. There is much discussion in the medical community whether high insulin levels cause obesity or if obesity causes them. Whatever the case, insulin resistance closely follows.

When insulin is high in the blood, it means that glucose is being metabolized at a faster rate than normal. Blood glucose falls and you get low blood sugar, a condition that is fatal if left untreated. The human body knows that if blood sugar is depleted, then bodily functions begin to shut down. This is why it forms a tolerance to insulin in order to survive. But if the body becomes too resistant to insulin, how will glucose be transported into the cells? The pancreas needs to produce even more insulin for the same effect to happen and you end up with a vicious cycle that is at the heart of diabetes.

High insulin leads to insulin resistance which in turn leads to higher insulin secretion. Type 1 diabetics are prescribed insulin because their bodies are incapable of producing it. Without regular insulin treatments, they will begin to waste away because no glucose energy is being delivered to cells. The kidney tries to get rid of the excess glucose through urination. Type 2 diabetics are given insulin treatments because they suffer from insulin resistance. This is a first line defense, though there have been cases of people treating their diabetes purely through diet. Over time, insulin resistance goes down if the body experiences fewer insulin spikes.

Insulin and insulin resistance are what make type 2 diabetes a chronic disease, to begin with. Insulin resistance is the result of a diet that is high in sugar and refined carbs. This diet is responsible for creating the high insulin levels that make up prediabetic conditions and the beginning of obesity. Obesity and diabetes are related diseases because in both cases, the high insulin levels lead to fat storage.

Common Misconceptions of Diabetes

1. **Sugar doesn't cause diabetes. It is genetic.**

The simplest answer to this is that yes, sugar doesn't cause diabetes in of itself. We already discussed that type 1 diabetes is genetic, while type 2 diabetes is a combination of genetic and lifestyle factors. There is without a scientific doubt, a causal relationship between sugar and insulin resistance. If you gorge on sugar, I guarantee that you will either develop some form of insulin resistance or fatty liver disease. You can have both of these conditions and still not be considered diabetic. That is, you have normal blood glucose levels. You will, however, be overweight and likely suffer from an increased risk of cardiovascular disease.

2. **I have to be overweight to be diabetic or being overweight causes diabetes.**

Again, being obese is closely associated with type 2 diabetes because both are involved with insulin resistance, but it doesn't mean that being overweight causes diabetes. Conversely, you could have a healthy BMI range and still have elevated levels of blood glucose. Diabetes is a complex disease and it varies on a case-by-case basis. Someone who is genetically predisposed to diabetes may have an excellent diet but still, suffer from diabetic conditions. Of course, a good diet will help in treating the disease but does not exclude the possibility of high blood sugar. That being said, if someone is overweight, they are likely eating tons of sugar and processed foods, because these two things are known to directly cause weight gain. An overweight person may very well be on their way to developing diabetes without fully knowing it.

3. **If I have diabetes, then I have to take insulin.**

This is only true for type 1 diabetes. If you have type 2 diabetes, you don't need insulin per se, but it can be prescribed to you by a doctor. The right diet may be all that you need, but this also varies. It is best to first speak with your doctor about available treatments. This will all depend on your current blood glucose levels and the overall progression of the disease. If you get diagnosed early and start leading a healthy lifestyle, you are less likely to need insulin with type 2 diabetes.

4. **Only older people have to care about getting diabetes.**

This is patently false. Juvenile diabetes is one of the most common for type 1 diabetes. Type 2 diabetes among children and adolescents is also on the rise. For many people who are genetically predisposed, there is no age where they suddenly have to start worrying about getting the disease. Don't let age be an excuse for not watching what you eat. People who do develop diabetes later in life tend to go from prediabetic conditions to full-on diabetes over time. People aren't simply born with insulin resistance, it is developed over time.

5. **I can't eat sugar if I am diabetic.**

If you follow an adequate diet and manage your diabetes, occasionally eating a sugary sweet will not cause inordinate harm. Your doctor will also tell you to avoid sugar the best you can. The tradeoff is largely up to you. How much are you willing to indulge versus how much risk are you willing to take. The risk is low if you are managing the disease regularly. Just be careful with binge eating, and definitely don't have your occasional sugary snacks in close proximity.

6. **I can't eat carbs if I am diabetic.**

Unlike with sugar, not all carbs are inherently evil. Refined carbs like flour, pasta, bread, cake, waffles, cookies, and so on are to be avoided. The low-carb diet is effective at treating diabetes because it lowers insulin resistance over time. Refined carbs are highly processed foods and lose the natural antidotes that counteract insulin secretion like fiber. Refined carbs are mechanically processed to be finer and finer. The finer the flour, the easier it is absorbed into the bloodstream. This is what leads to large insulin spikes. In contrast, coarse grains full in fiber and trace amounts of protein and fat are slowly absorbed. Sometimes, it is recommendable to forgo carbohydrates altogether, but not always necessary. The low carb diet still allows you to occasionally eat whole wheat bread and potatoes, for example. It's not that you can't eat carbs, you just shouldn't be eating a lot of them. And especially none of the refined variety. Eat as natural as you can.

7. **Diabetes isn't that serious.**

I think the misconception about diabetes not being a serious disease stems from how treatable it is. If you manage the disease, it may appear like nothing is wrong with you. You may not experience any of the symptoms from glucotoxicity and think that it is no big deal. The fact of the matter is that diabetes kills people. Diabetes and high blood glucose related disorders kill millions each year globally and are on the rise. I already went over the possible complications of the disease, so I doubt you buy into diabetes not being a serious disease. What I will say though, is that diabetes is a manageable disease. If you take the necessary steps, there is no reason why you can't live a long healthy life while still being diabetic. But it is largely up to you to take those steps. Nobody else can take them for you.

Diabetes Diagnosis and Blood Sugar Management

Today, we have more sophisticated methods for diagnosing diabetes. In the past, the disease could only be guesstimated by the signs and symptoms present. This would mean looking for the presence of sugar in the urine and noting how often the patient went to the bathroom. Weight loss and extreme hunger were also tell-tale signs that something is wrong. We know now that diabetes is a disorder of blood glucose and it can be diagnosed by simply measuring the concentration of glucose in the blood.

The most straightforward way to measure blood glucose is by using a home glucose monitoring device where you must prick your finger on a lancet onto a test strip. Different devices have their own methodologies, but they all follow a similar protocol. Non-invasive meters have been in the works for years now, with not a single suitable product ever penetrating the market. As of writing, no such device has passed FDA guidelines, so I do not recommend looking at non-invasive products. The standard method gets a little getting used to, but it is your safest bet for monitoring blood glucose. It should still be noted that non-invasive devices are a part of active research and a solution that works just as good as finger pricking may be achieved in the future. To get the most accurate read of your blood glucose, perform the test immediately after waking up and before eating any meals. This measures your fasting blood glucose rate. Since you eat several meals throughout the day, the fasting blood glucose rate gives you a better idea of how glucose is concentrated in the blood without it being mistaken by blood sugar spikes from eating.

Your doctor will likely perform more advanced tests every three to six months to see if you are making any progress. The test doctors use is called hemoglobin A1C. It measures a protein found in red blood cells and the amount of glucose attached to it. This test is usually given as a percentage in the United States and as a measurement in other countries. The breakdown of hemoglobin A1C is as follows: an A1C score less than 5.7 percent is considered healthy, a score in between 5.7 and 6.4 percent is considered prediabetic, and anything greater than 6.5 is considered diabetic. It is important that you know this score and that you keep track of it over time. Doubtless, your doctor will do this for you, but I encourage you to be proactive when managing the disease yourself. These are your numbers, so to speak.

Fasting blood sugar of less than 100 mg/dL is considered healthy. A fasting blood sugar level between 100 and 125 mg/dL is considered prediabetic. Anything above 126 mg/dL is considered diabetic. Another test used by doctors to measure the fasting glucose is called the oral glucose tolerance test. You fast the entire night and come into the lab to drink a syrupy substance. The test is designed to measure how your body handles a sudden consumption of sugar. Two hours after taking the drink, your blood sugar is measured again. If after two hours your blood glucose is lower than 140 mg/dL, then you are in the normal range. A blood glucose level between 140 and 199 mg/dl is considered prediabetic and anything at or above 200 mg/dL is considered fully diabetic.

Knowing these numbers is the key to knowing how well you are managing your diabetes.

When it comes to home testing, you will want to take multiple measurements throughout the day. Usually, the intervals at which you test your blood sugar will be designated by your doctor or healthcare professional but to give a general idea, they should be taken before and after meals and before and after waking. It is very important to take a measurement right after waking up to get your fasting blood glucose rate. Next, you are going to want to take another measurement before lunch and dinner and again two hours after. Finally, take another measurement before going to bed.

Also, take measurements before you engage in strenuous exercise. Blood sugar can fall quickly when exercising so make sure that it is high enough to perform the workout. If you are diabetic and your blood sugar is less than 100 mg/dL before exercise, it is best not to perform it right away. Instead, eat a small meal or even take glucose tablets if you have them available. A serving of fruit or snack bar should be enough to get blood sugar above this level. Avoid exercising on a completely empty stomach. If your blood glucose is in between 100 and 250 mg/dL, then you are in the sweet spot for exercise. However, if the blood sugar rate is above 250 mg/dL, you are advised not to exercise. If you do exercise with a high blood sugar level, you risk a serious complication called ketoacidosis.

Note that these are general guidelines for when to check blood sugar. Check in with your doctor for the recommended frequency. It will vary from person to person and from type 1 diabetics and type 2 diabetics. Additionally, your doctor will set you up with a target range for blood glucose level. The number of factors that may affect this range is myriad. First, you have the type of diabetes, the severity of the disease, how old you are, how long you've been diagnosed with diabetes for, whether or not you are pregnant, and your overall health. According to the Mayo Clinic, your blood sugar before meals should be between 80 and 120 mg/dL if you are under the age of 59. If you are above the age of 60, the Mayo Clinic recommends a range between 100 and 140 mg/dL assuming you have no other medical conditions.

More general guidelines given by the American Diabetes Association are that blood sugar should be between 80 and 130 mg/dL before meals and less than 180 mg/dL two hours after meals. If your numbers vary drastically from these, you may need to call your emergency numbers. Symptoms of hypoglycemia usually don't occur before blood glucose is below 50 mg/dL. But don't feel like you have to wait for the symptoms to appear to check your glucose. If your levels are below your target range, you should eat something. Probably some form of carbohydrate.

You will want to check your glucose more frequently when you feel symptoms of hypoglycemia coming. Other times, you will want to check are during illness and times of stress. If you are suddenly more active or suddenly less active, your blood glucose can vary. Also, check more frequently if you have recently changed insulin or other medications.

Monitoring your blood glucose is important because it is a definite way to diagnose hypoglycemia and hyperglycemia. Note that if the concentration of blood glucose is either too low or too high, it could be a medical emergency. You may be off put by the amount of effort it takes to take multiple daily measurements. They are worth it and can potentially save your life. The more you make a habit of taking daily measurements the less of a burden they will feel like.

Chapter 2: Diabetic Diet: The Low-Carb Diet

Obesity and diabetes are both associated with insulin resistance. For the type 2 diabetic, they can no longer make effective use of normal doses of insulin, and so, their blood sugar doesn't go down to normal levels. In the obese person, insulin resistance is marked by the bodies tendency to store fat. If glucose isn't being used up as energy, it gets converted into triglycerides. This is especially true in the form of organ fat or visceral fat. A person with an otherwise healthy BMI may still suffer from what is termed "central obesity" or the culmination of visceral fat that results in fat bellies. If insulin resistance plays such a damning role in these conditions, the logical first step of treatment is to lower it. One possible way to do just that is through the low-carb diet. Carbohydrates directly cause blood glucose to go up after ingested, which in turn, causes insulin to be secreted by the beta cells in the pancreas. After a time, the body gets used to the insulin response and requires more of it for the same amount of energy to be used. In other words, the more carbs one is eating, the higher they are raising their insulin resistance.

In practice, the story is a little more complex than that as you can probably imagine. There are other sources of insulin secretion in the body, like the incretin hormones found in the stomach that release insulin after the protein is ingested. Though simplified as it is, the model of insulin resistance presented here gives a strong argument for adopting a low-carb diet. Consider the potential drawbacks of such diet versus the potential gains. On the one hand, you get to eat less comfort food, but on the other, you gain the possibility of lowering your insulin resistance. If it sounds too good to be true, then you should read on and decide for yourself. The low-carb diet has been shown to work both in experimental studies and from anecdotal evidence.

I believe that the low-carb diet is the diet that has been used throughout the world for centuries. Before agriculture was a thing, it is likely that our ancestors subsisted on high-protein, high-fat diets. Early humans hunted for animal meat and fats. They likely drank the blood of animals as well. Their carbs probably came from foraged berries, tubers, and seeds and nuts. What I just described is what modern dieters call the "Paleo" or Paleolithic diet. Eating food that is all natural and fresh is ultimately better than food that is highly processed. Whether one tastes better than the other is up to debate, but the taste should never come before health.

As early as the 19th century, people started to realize how modern life was essentially making us fat. In 1863, well into the industrial age, an obese undertaker named William Banting designed one of the earliest versions of the low-carb diet. Banting was dissatisfied with the state of his weight. At 66, the five foot five man weighed some 202 pounds, which isn't really bad in today's standards. Banting discovered that eating less and exercising more did little to bring his weight down. Eventually, on the recommendation of a surgeon, he tried cutting out all breads, butter, milk, sugar, beer, and potatoes. As you can probably tell, this is a cut and dry low-carb approach. Back then, these foods were less processed than today, and his previous diet is more akin to a low-refined carb diet. In his pamphlet titled *Letter on Corpulence Addressed to the Public*, he admits that he indulged in those non-refined more than what the average man probably would.

A Calorie Is not a Calorie

Over the course of one year, Banting lost a whopping 46 pounds by simply changing what he ate. The dirge behind many diets today is that people lose a few pounds only to regain them all back later. This initial loss in weight can be attributed to a little mechanism in the body called homeostasis. The body burns a set number of calories every day needed to sustain life. Things like temperature regulation, tissue repair, and growth all cost caloric energy, which is primarily derived from glucose as the main energy source. The amount of energy your body burns by simply staying alive is called the basal metabolic rate and is responsible for 95 percent of all energy expenditure. The other 5 percent is attributed to things like exercise and going about your daily activities.

What happens when you start cutting calories or going on a caloric restriction diet is that the body takes in less energy but burns the same amount. Since our bodies are smart and designed to withstand times of famine, they do a really clever thing when a drop in calories is detected. First, they shut down non-vital energy expenditure. Things like temperate regulation can simply be cut out because you can still live while being cold. The basal metabolic rate goes down, and what little energy does come in is used sparsely. If you were eating a diet of 3,000 calories a day, your body could be burning some 2,800 just on its own. If you then lowered calorie consumption to a mere 1,800 a day, your body detects the change and goes into starvation mode. In an attempt to conserve energy, the basal metabolic falls to just 1,500. In both cases, you are at a caloric surplus, despite thinking you are on a deficit! This is why Banting could not lose weight by simply eating less and exercising more. What's more, many caloric restrictive diets are miserable to stay on. They are tough on the body and cause many people to simply stop the diet. Someone who starts eating less will be cold all the time and suffer from poor concentration and mood swings. They feel tired all the time. Worst of all, they will suffer from hunger. Hunger is probably the ultimate diet killer. It is unpleasant and just feels wrong. Your own body coaxes you to eat more food. And since food is readily available in our lives, hunger is easily stopped.

Homeostasis is a mechanism that strives to keep things stable. If your weight goes a little bit up because you consume more calories, your metabolism rises to match the excess energy. Over time, your weight comes back to normal and your metabolism slows. And if you eat too little, the initial weight loss goes back to pre-dieting numbers. There seems to be the existence of a "set weight" that the body returns to. Set weight theory is contested in the medical community (some say it has a little scientific basis) but the hormonal regulation of weight is more accepted. That is, our weight is regulated by the interactions of different hormones in the body. Insulin, for example, acts as the receptor that tells cells when to use up glucose for energy. It is not that obese people lack self-control, but that their hormones are out of whack. Remember that high insulin levels cause insulin resistance and that the more glucose that is not being used gets converted into visceral fat. Fat equals weight gain. Insulin and insulin resistance effectively bring up the set weight, causing people to gain even more weight in the long run. This type of weight gain is difficult to reduce, and it only gets harder as time goes by. No matter how much dieting and exercising you do, you will not bring down that set weight because your diet isn't affecting the root cause. The root cause is insulin.

For decades, people have pushed the idea that calories in must be lower than calories out if you want to lose weight. But as we have seen with homeostasis, that simply is not true. If calories in are reduced, calories out will adapt to the change and drop as well. You reap zero benefits for all the troubles of restricting your calories. This way of thinking is rooted in the myth that calories are the irreducible unit of energy and that all calories are the same. Among the three macronutrients of protein, carbohydrates, and dietary fat, all three cause different hormonal responses in the body.

Proteins are broken down into their respective amino acids and are recombined to create new hormones, muscle, and tissue. Dietary fat is converted into fatty acids. Carbohydrates (chains of sugars) are either used directly in the form of glucose or in the case of things like fructose, are converted into glucose first. We already know that sugar and refined carbohydrates cause insulin to go up. The glucose from the ingested carbohydrate will either be used for energy or stored in body fat.

Additional benefits of a low-carb diet

Besides the obvious benefits of lowering blood glucose and insulin levels, low-carb diets have a myriad of hidden benefits that you can only experience by making the switch.

1. **Increased Energy Levels**

    The low-carb diets have you feeling full of energy. You won't feel lousy after every meal. Many people are put off by the low-carb diet because they fear that they won't get any energy. This is a common misconception and is associated with the initial "lull" you might feel after you make the switch. Your body will not be used to the diet and the beginning is rough. Your body will look for additional sugar to burn as energy, but since very little is coming in, it will convert available glycogen stores. Eventually, your body switches to burning fat for energy instead. This not only fosters weight loss, but it gives you a constant source of energy. Sugar crashes will be a thing of yesterday

2. **Lower Anxiety and Depression**

The link between sugar, refined carbohydrates, and depression has long been talked about. Sugar is a highly addictive substance that can coax sweet receptors in the brain to associate it with rewards. Just desserts make the brain crave more and more of the white substance. Its addictiveness has been compared to that of hard drugs. Any serious addiction can have depressive effects, and not just the ones derived from drugs.

Cutting sugar from your diet breaks the addiction. You probably think you aren't addicted to sugar but that is difficult to tell. Almost every processed food now contains sugar. Even innocuous food items like sauces and other condiments may contain traces of sugar. So-called "healthy" breakfast cereals are notorious offenders, right beside fruit juice. Some of these products contain high-fructose corn syrup, a sugar product made from processed corn. Corn syrup with high fructose is even worse than sugar because it is almost pure fructose.

Comfort food is more sinister than you might think. We tend to eat sugary things when we are sad, stressed, or anxious because they make us feel good. That good feeling is essentially a pleasure response from your sweetness receptors, but it is a temporary high. And how do addicts supplant temporary highs? By eating more of the stuff. The end result is that you feel miserable from the sugar crash, and whatever was making you sad, stressed, or anxious in the first place is still there.

3. **Better Sleep**

People who go on low-carb diets report having better sleep than those who do not. The first few nights might be rough because your body isn't used to the diet. But after the initial lull, it is smooth sailing and deep sleeping. The exact mechanisms of diet on sleep are not well understood, but some studies have shown that low-carb dieters spend more time in the deep-sleep stage. Anecdotal evidence echoes these results among those who take low-carb diets. They experience better sleep, reduced insomnia, and better wakefulness in the morning.

4. **May Protect Against Cancer**

Once a cell turns cancerous, the tumor has an insatiable hunger for resources. This is bad news for people with high blood sugar, as there are vast quantities of the energy supply for the tumor to feed on. Many cancer cells are equipped with insulin receptors that also benefit from a high insulin level in the blood. A low-carb diet effectively reduces both insulin and blood sugar, making it a potential treatment for those at risk of getting cancer.

5. **Overcome Cravings**

A low-carb diet is fuller and is a one-way ticket off the sugar craving rollercoaster. If you stick with the diet, your cravings for comfort food will drop. You will feel fuller after meals and you will think twice before picking up something sugary just for the energy boost. If you have a sweet tooth, the more time you go abstaining from sugar, the less you will want to go back to your sugary ways. As you will learn later in this book, a low-carb diet doesn't have to be one that tastes bad. It might not always be sweet, but you certainly won't be eating cardboard for the rest of your days.

6. **Lower Risk of Heart Disease**

Another consequence of the low-fat diet is that higher importance was put on the carbohydrate. Traditionally the bottom or foundation of the pyramid consisted of bread, pasta, grains, cereals, starchy vegetables, and so forth. It's more common now for the bottom row to be dedicated to water. The war against fat created an artificial glut for carbohydrates. Carbohydrates directly cause blood glucose to go up and start the insulin resistance cycle. It is no wonder that obesity and diabetes rose during the national campaign against fat.

A low-carb diet, while high in animal proteins and fat, can lower the cardiovascular risk far better than a low-fat diet. Why is this? Because it reverses all of the mechanisms that make diabetes such a cardiovascular risk. It lowers blood glucose, diminishing the role of glucotoxicity on the blood vessels. It lowers visceral fat in the organs that cause central obesity.

But isn't a diet high in fats also high in cholesterol? Yes, these diets are high in cholesterol. Think eggs, a major cholesterol source in our diet. While cholesterol is high, it doesn't directly transfer to blood-cholesterol. While saturated fats raise LDL or bad cholesterol, they simultaneously raise HDL or good cholesterol. In recent years, saturated fat and high-fat diets have been accepted as healthy. Diets that are high in carbohydrates (especially refined ones including sugar) are now associated with a greater heart disease risk than high-fat diets.

7. **Benefits for the Brain**

Even on a low-carb diet, the body uses a process called glycogenesis to create new glucose. Glycogenesis can either convert glycol found in stored fat into glucose or amino acids formed from proteins. Additionally, through the process of ketosis, the body can supply energy to the brain derived from ketones. If you are worried about your brain getting enough energy, you can rest assured that a low-carb diet will supply your precious thinking muscle with all the energy it needs. That is, of course, if you eat at your recommended calorie intake.

Is there a difference between a brain supplied by pure glucose and a brain supplied by ketones or glucose derived from fat? The effects on brain function are little understood, but some preliminary studies have found hidden benefits. Studies in older mice using a ketogenic low-carb diet have resulted in improved cognitive function, for example. What's more, a condition called congenital hyperinsulinism has been successfully treated by a ketogenic low-carb diet. Congenital hyperinsulinism is characterized by high insulin which leads to extreme hypoglycemia that can cause brain damage.

Those who suffer from type 2 diabetes are at an increased risk for Alzheimer's disease. A recent study even goes as far as to say that Alzheimer's is actually the final stage of type 2 diabetes. The insulin levels that a type 2 diabetic produces to counteract insulin resistance is poisonous to the brain. What can be done to stop the progression of Alzheimer's among those who are at risk? Well, one study found that older, at-risk patients improved their memory by switching to a low-carb diet in little as six weeks.

Types of Low-Carb Diets

So far, you have heard tons of information about the low-carb diet, but you may probably want specifics. I have already mentioned two possible variations in the previous section and those are the ketogenic and the Paleolithic diets. Low-carb diets come in different flavors, but they all do more or less the same thing. Pick whichever one is best for you and your goals. I will provide a general outline of some of the most popular low-carb diets below.

Low Carb High Fat (LCHF)

The low carb high-fat diet is one of the most effective at treating diabetes. Carbs are kept at a minimum, meanwhile, protein consumption is moderate and fat consumption is high. All forms of dairy are allowed including the most dreaded whole milk and cheeses. This diet works both at lowering weight and insulin levels, the perfect combination for fighting obesity and diabetes at once. Modern fat propaganda has branded all dietary fat sources as killers. However, the truth about dietary fat is more nuanced than that. Heart disease is the number one ailment that the health community cites when it comes to the dangers of fat. The same can be said for the championing of low-fat diets starting in the 1970s when America was suffering from increased incidence of heart disease.

Healthy fats come from fatty cuts of meat, fish, whole eggs, and whole dairy sources. Nuts high in fat and avocados are also high-fat favorites. Vegetable oils and butter can be used when cooking all your meals. Cooking with oil is both better tasting and healthy in fat. Proteins are your standard run of the mill meats and dairy. Most proteins will be good for your diet, so you can pick and choose your favorites. Though since you also want to target high-fat counts, avoid very lean meats. If you like poultry, always keep the skin on for a boost in fat.

The carbohydrate content in these diets may vary. Extremely low carbohydrate counts are not recommended. Sugar is refined carbs which are not allowed. For a very strict LCHF diet, keep your carbohydrate count below 20 grams a day. For a moderate LCHF diet, use around 20 – 50 grams of carb. And for a liberal LCHF diet, use 50 – 100 grams.

Since LCHF is strict on carbohydrates, you will probably want to avoid most fruits

Ketogenic Diet

The ketogenic diet is basically a very strict LCHF diet. Carb consumption is extremely discouraged because the emphasis is on fat burning. Like with the LCHF and other low-carb diets, there is a greater emphasis on whole foods. No sugar, no refined carbs, and little fruit.

As such, the keto diet is considered "extreme," especially for diabetics. Twenty grams of carbohydrates may be derived from just one cup of starchy vegetables, for example. For a ketogenic diet to work the way it is intended, the dieter must stick completely with the diet guidelines and their targeted macronutrient consumption. It really is a "go big or go home" type of scenario. Consequently, you can't eat most fruits, and definitely no carbohydrate greater than 20g. Keto diets work by putting the body into a metabolic state called "ketosis". Anyone who wants to use this diet seriously needs to first understand how ketosis develops.

When the body runs out of glucose to use as energy, it instead turns to fat. Ketones, short for "ketone bodies", are the by-products of fat being broken down for energy. As blood glucose levels go down, so does insulin since there is no need to bind to cell receptors and let the glucose in. The body then looks for an alternative food source, namely fat. Chances are that your body has undergone ketosis in your daily life already. Fasting for long periods of time like during sleep may deplete glucose and glycogen stores leading to a state of ketosis. The same can be said for strenuous exercise, starvation, and of course, when eating a low-carb diet.

These ketones are capable of powering virtually every part of your body. You don't have to worry about your brain struggling because it can directly use ketone bodies for energy. Just like with blood sugar, it is possible for excess ketones to build up in the blood. Ketone levels are usually quantified using millimoles per liter (mmol/L). A negative level of ketones is less than .6 mmol/L, a low to moderate level is between .6 and 1.5 mmol/L, a high ketone level is from 1.6 to 3.0 mmol/L and a very high ketone level is above 3.0 mmol.

There are various ways to test for ketone bodies. You can pee on a strip to test ketones in urine. These strips are inexpensive at readily available but tend to be inaccurate the longer you are in ketosis. You can also use the same blood glucose meter you use to test for blood sugar. All you need is a different test strip that works specifically for ketones in the blood. This method is very accurate, but the strips tend to be expensive. One final way to test for ketones is to use a breathing device like a Ketonic that tests the amount of a certain ketone released in your breath.

Besides testing these levels manually, there are tell-tale signs that indicate that you are in a state of ketosis. Unfortunately, since one of the ketone bodies called acetone leaves the body through the breath, those in ketosis suffer from bad breath. This is easily counteracted by dental hygiene products and sugar-free gum. You will also feel an initial lull as your blood glucose begins to drop. You will experience all the same symptoms from hypoglycemia. If you exercise regularly, you will experience an initial depreciation in your athletic ability as the main energy source in muscles called glycogen is depleted. When your body successfully goes into ketosis though, you will experience increased energy levels and a reduced appetite.

As a diabetic going on the ketogenic diet, there is an increased concern with ketone levels because they can lead to a condition called ketoacidosis. This condition is mostly associated with type 1 diabetics because they lack the ability to create new insulin on their own. In any case, talk with your doctor before starting this type of diet.

Low Carb Paleo

A paleo diet short for paleolithic focuses on all natural, non-processed foods that typically early humans would be able to eat. Because of this extra restriction, you cannot eat all forms of dairy, legumes, and grains. Early humans were not domesticating cattle, and they certainly weren't starting out in agriculture. Most starchy vegetables are also out of the picture. Practitioners of paleo will tell you that white potatoes are a big no, no and those sweet potatoes are totally fine.

Though a premium is given on protein, you can't eat anything that is overly processed. Nine times out of then this means that you have to eat fresh from the butcher or choose organic bee. Free-range is also a popular choice. You can't eat most sausages, bacon, and packaged deli meats. You can enjoy all types of fresh fish, eggs and lean cuts of poultry, pork, and beef. All non-starchy vegetables are for grabs including peppers, broccoli, spinach, and kale. You can also enjoy every variety of fruit and nuts. Most of your carbohydrate will be in the form of fruits and non-starchy vegetables.

Atkins 40 Diet

The Atkins diet was popularized by a physician named Robert Atkins to promote weight loss. The first iteration of the diet consisted of highly controlled carbohydrate consumption, high protein, and fats. For the most part, dieters were allowed to choose their macronutrients however they wanted as long as they emphasize low carb consumption. When it was first brought to the mainstream in the 1970s, it got a bad rap from the health community because they believed it put dieters at a greater risk of cardiovascular disease. Many believed Atkins as well as other low-carb diets to be "fad diets" rather than hardcore, evidence-based weight loss treatments. Unfortunately, the bad reputation behind this diet has stuck around into modern times. When it was first introduced, people did lose weight like on any other diet. However, they would eventually gain most of the weight back even while on the diet. Since then, the diet has been revised to correct for high meat content, which may have caused dieters to regain weight. The diet has been through multiple iterations over the years. A solid version of it exists today called the Atkins 40, denoting the number of carbs you are allowed to eat daily.

In addition to 40g of carbohydrate, you are also allowed to eat 3 servings of protein a day and 2 – 3 servings of fat from added fats. Each serving of protein is between 4 and 6 ounces, and each serving of fat is about one tablespoon. If you split the number of carbs during each meal, you can have three meals with 10g carbs and two 5g snacks throughout the day, or however you wish. Fifteen grams of these carbohydrates should come from 6-8 servings of "foundational vegetables". This includes both starchy and non-starchy varieties. Note that these grams are calculated as "net carbs" which are total carbohydrate minus fiber minus sugar alcohols. The other 25g of carbohydrate can come from various sources that you pick. These can be from dairy, alcohol, bread, pasta, you name it. The only things you can't eat are refined carbs and sugar.

Banting Diet

The Banting diet is a name given to a general class of low-carb diets that follow the teachings of William Banting and his success in losing weight. Again, the Banting diet follows the familiar mantra of eating all-natural foods and limiting sugar and refined carbs. The calories lost from carbohydrates should be given to fat, rather than protein. This includes buying fatty cuts of meat. Instead of saying to completely eliminate refined carbs, the Banting diet simply says to "limit consumption". Carb consumption should be no more than 50 or 60g a day, with the majority of them coming from non-refined carbohydrates. The final breakdown of macronutrients is 10 – 15% calories from carbohydrates, 15 – 25% percent calories from proteins, and 60 – 70% calories from fat. As you can see, your consumption of fat will largely determine how much protein and carbs you consume.

Low Carb Diet Guidelines

The number of calories you consume on the low-carb diet will depend on your age, gender, current weight, and how active you are. If are you looking to lose weight, you might want to eat a little less as well. Generally, the low-carb diet allows you to lose weight even at a caloric surplus because you will be burning more fat than glucose. If you are overweight or have a high BMI, you may consider eating slightly less.

Here are some general caloric guidelines for all age groups. Note that your doctor will probably give you a caloric target range. Low-carb diets are safe both for the elderly and for children below 18.

Children

Young children are very active by nature and may need high-calorie counts relative to their size. They are also at an increased risk of eating junk food. Food companies tend to target young children more than any age group when it comes to selling sugary refined carbs. Children also naturally gravitate towards things that are sweet, like candy and fruit juices. If your child is diabetic, you will have to cut their access to such foods. Since they are underage, you will have to manage their diabetes for them.

Caloric Requirements

Children aged 4 through 13 need around 1,200 to 1,600 calories if they lead a sedentary lifestyle, 1,400 to 2,000 if they are moderately active, and 1,400 to 2,200 if they are active. Moderately active children exert physical activity equivalent of 1.5 to 3 miles a day and active children greater than the equivalent of 3 miles a day.

Adults

Adults are at an increased risk of sedentary lifestyles than children especially among those who have office jobs. However, their caloric needs vary more depending on weight. The low-carb diet is a favorite among those looking to lose weight and those who suffer from gluten intolerances.

Caloric Requirements

To calculate the caloric requirement for adults, you will first have to calculate the basal metabolic rate (BMR). Note that it is tricky to do this outside of a laboratory setting. And even then, the BMR is constantly shifting to meet caloric intake. You can calculate a pretty good estimate using an online formula. Usually, these formulas take into account your gender, body fat percentage, and daily physical activity through work and exercise. You can also ask your doctor for the most substantive testing.

It is very important that you know how much calories you should be eating. If all else fails, you can use the following guidelines to "eye-ball" your caloric requirement.

1,200 to 1,600 calories a day if
- You are a small woman who exercises
- Small to medium-sized woman who wants to lose weight
- Medium-sized woman sedentary woman

1,600 to 2,000 a day if
- Large woman who wants to lose weight
- Small man at a healthy weight
- Medium-sized sedentary man
- Medium-sized or large man who wants to lose weight

2,000 to 2,400 a day if
- Medium-sized or large man who works a physically demanding job or works out regularly
- Large man at a healthy weight
- Medium-sized or large woman who works a physically demanding job or works out

Seniors

The elderly stand to benefit from low-carb diets because they get their share of healthy fats, proteins, and little to no sugar and refined carbs. The elderly may have additional sodium and fiber requirements, so carbohydrates should include plenty of leafy greens and other vegetables. Ample sodium can be derived from bone broths. Seniors also benefit from the many nutrients in a moderately protein rich diet. These include iron, B12, and vitamin D.

Seniors may use the above adult caloric guidelines.

Customizing your low-carb diet

Once you know your daily caloric needs and pick a diet, you can begin customizing your diet to fit your tastes. There are many readily available meal plans online for low-carb, but you should also learn how to calculate energy content and macros on your own. For example, if your daily caloric intake is 2,200, you will have to split your food along the correct macro ratios. Carbohydrates and proteins both contain 4 calories per gram while the much denser dietary fats contain 9 calories per gram. Since low-carb diets are high in fats, you will be eating less food in terms of gross weight. For simplicity sake, we will use net carbs to calculate calories.

LCHF Ratios

LCHF rations depend on what version of the diet you are going with. A moderate LCHF calls for 20 – 50 grams of carbohydrate.

2,200 caloric needs

50g net carbs = 200 calories (9%)
140g protein = 560 calories (25%)
161g fats = 1,452 calories (66%)

Ketogenic Ratios

Keto macros are a little more involved and depend on your physical properties as well as your activity level. Twenty grams of carbs is generally considered the sweet spot for inducing ketosis. Add 10 – 20g if you are an athlete with high carbohydrate needs.

Protein is calculated by first finding out your fat content. You need to know your weight as well as your body fat percentage.

Total fat = bodyweight x body fat percentage.

Calculate your lean body mass

Lean body mass = 100 – body fat percentage X 100
Divide by 100 to get your muscle weight

Muscle weight = lean body mass / 100

Now find your total lean muscle mass:

Weight X muscle weight = lean mass

Here is an example assuming a weight of 160 lbs and body fat of 20%

160 pounds X .20 = 32 body fat lbs
100 - .20 X 100 = 80% body mass
80 / 100 = .80 muscle weight
160 X 0.80 = 128 lean mass

Then you figure out your protein needs, multiply lean mass by protein grams.

128 X .8 = 102

Those .8 grams of protein per pound of lean mass are only a recommendation. You can use anywhere from .7 – 1 gram of protein per pound.

The rest of your macros should go to fat

20g net carbs = 80 calories (3%)
102g protein = 408 calories (18%)
193g fat = 1737 calories (79%)

Low-carb Paleo Ratios

Here is an example for a low to moderate carb paleo diet.

83g net carbs = 330 calories (15%)
165g protein = 660 calories (30%)
158g fat = 1,430 calories (65%)

Atkins 40 Ratios

The Atkins 40 is based around a number of servings rather than strict macro counting. The only set requirement is 40g of carbohydrate. Next is 3 servings of 4 – 6 ounces of protein. Finally, you can have 2 to 4 servings of fat each of 1 tablespoon. This is calorically dense, both from the protein and fat sources. There are 15 grams of fat in a single teaspoon. If you convert 2 tablespoon servings into grams, you get about 90.

40g net carbs = 160 calories
339g protein = 1,356
90g fat = 810 calories

Using the bare minimum values, we get a net of 2,326 calories which is higher than our target 2,200. You can lower this by losing either one serving of fat or protein.

Banting Diet Ratios

The Banting diet has straightforward rations, 10 – 15% carb, 15 to 25% protein, and 60-70% fats.

82 net carb = 330 calories (15%)

137g = 550 calories (25%)

146g = 1,320 calories (60%)

Once you understand how to count your macros, you will able to customize your diets with whatever food that fit those macros. Caloric content of popular foods are readily available online, so get counting!

Chapter 3: The Diabetic Food List

As mentioned in the previous chapter, not every calorie is the same. There are two main effects from food metabolism that diabetics need to be on the lookout for. The first is blood glucose rise and the second are insulin spikes. Glucose response can be measured by using a scale called the glycemic index. The glycemic index measures the effect that carbohydrates have on blood sugar two hours after consumption. A glycemic index of 100 denotes the max on the scale. A score of 100 is pure glucose, and any carb food will score below that. The glycemic index gives a good indication of what you should and should not eat. Avoid foods that are higher than 70, and closely moderate foods that are between 55 and 69. Anything below 55 is considered good; the lower the better. The glycemic index is useful, however, it isn't perfect. It doesn't measure insulin response, which is the other effect that diabetics need to manage. Contrary to popular belief, all foods increase insulin not just carbohydrates. But since carbs are made up of chains of sugars, they have a significant effect on blood glucose, and therefore, insulin as well. Foods that score low on the glycemic index (less than 55) are called low-glycemic foods. Low-glycemic foods are a safe bet for diabetics, and those that score high should only be eaten in moderation.

Though even on a low-carb diet, there are certain protein and fat sources you might want to avoid as well.

Carbohydrates

You already know that you are supposed to limit these in your intake. But, I think it is a good practice to go over the individual foods to clean up any confusion. You will probably be curious to see how some carbs rank on the various indexes as well. A good rule of thumb is to avoid all processed foods. Basically, anything that comes pre-packaged. If you do have to eat from packaged food, beware of high-fructose corn syrup in the ingredients list. Fructose is basically just sugar given a fancy name. It is not corn, period. You will have to read the ingredient list carefully. Sometimes, added sugar is masqueraded under a number of different names. These include dextrose, dextrin, maltol, maltose, saccharose, agave nectar, and several others. For an exhaustive list of these substitutes, you will have to do your own research. Added sugar has a tendency to hide in plain sight; this is why you should avoid packaged food altogether. Eating at restaurants also presents a problem because you can't always get the ingredients list. Sauces and fried foods are likely to contain sugar without you even knowing it.

White Flour
Glycemic index: 85

Flour is used in a myriad of high sugar, high processed carb-rich foods. The modern milling process grinds flour to such fine grains that they are instantly absorbed into the bloodstream upon ingestion, shooting blood glucose through the roof. It is not surprising that white flour is so high on the glycemic index. White flour gets its characteristic white color from a chemical bleaching process used to speed up aging. If the ingredients label doesn't list whether the flour is bleached or not, you can assume that it is bleached. Bleaching results in finer particles and the loss of trace amounts of other macronutrients and fiber. For this reason, unbleached flour is always superior. Unbleached flour also has a higher protein content which results in harder bread, but it is good for you relatively speaking.

Don't be fooled by the labels on white flour. Whether it is bleached or unbleached, it is still a refined grain. This means that the wheat kernel is stripped of the bran and the germ, leaving only the endosperm. There is no fiber, B-vitamins, or iron normally found in unrefined wheat.

Bottom Line: Avoid white flour in all its forms. If you must eat on a special occasion or the rare dessert, go for the unbleached variety. If you really like bread and wish to consume it without any guilt, there are several alternative and specialty flours that have a lower GI index. These include walnut flour, soy flour, almond flour, flaxseed, chickpea flour, and even coconut flour. Note that these alternatives tend to be on the expensive side.

Enriched Flour
Glycemic Index: 85+

If white flour is bad, enriched flour is worse. A refined flour is enriched when the nutrients it lost from the milling process are chemically added to the final product. While it is advertised as healthier than the pure white flour variety, it tends to score higher on the glycemic index. This is the epitome of processed food: first nutrients are removed through mechanical milling, then they are chemically added. Talk about a double whammy. Beware of this type of flour in your ingredient list. It is commonly found in flour tortillas products.

Bottom Line: Worse than regular flour, it should definitely be avoided. If you want the benefits from the added nutrients, whole wheat bread is a better option.

Whole Wheat Flour
Glycemic Index: 69

Whole wheat contains the entire kernel, and so is coarser than white flour grains. However, it still has a mid-range glycemic index of 69. Whole wheat flour is still refined but less so than white flour. You get the additional nutrients from the whole kernel and are slightly slower to digest than white flour. The terminology used on the ingredients list is a little confusing. If you don't see the word "whole" included, then it probably isn't whole wheat. Simply "what" or "grain" bread may not be made using the whole kernel. Additionally, sometimes, breads are listed as "whole grain". Whole grain simply means that the kernel can come from any grain, including oats, spelt, and barley. Some of those other grains score in the lower mid-range glycemic index and are better for you.

Bottom Line: Most whole wheat breads you buy at the store are still considered processed foods and are thus fast absorbing into the bloodstream. For that reason, they should be limited and certainly not consumed on a daily basis. While more nutritionally dense than white flour, whole wheat is still refined. A better alternative is to find whole wheat bread that is made from a stone mill, but good luck finding that at your local grocery store. If you are a home baker or if you shop at specialty stores, the sourdough process brings down the glycemic index. Authentic sourdough has a glycemic index of 53 and is a good option for those with a bread craving. Like all carbs in the low-carb diet, you still want to limit consumption to an occasional basis.

Sugary Baked Goods
Glycemic Index: 72 (Blueberry white flour muffin)

It goes without saying but sugary baked goods are a diabetics worst nightmare for blood glucose intake. Most of these products are derived from white flour and added sugar, high fructose corn syrup, and other sweeteners. The simple solution is to not eat these types of foods at all. Foods included in this category include all kinds of muffins, pies cakes, pancakes, pastries, sweet breads, crepes, etc. For some people, eating these foods is a natural response to stress and hardship in their daily lives. Unfortunately, they are fattening and cause insulin levels to soar. As with other sugary foods, they elicit a pleasure response in the brain making you want to crave them even more.

Bottom Line: Severely reduce or eliminate these foods from your diet. If you must eat them, look into diabetic alternatives and specialty foods. Again, this is a more expensive option but if you have a sweet tooth they are better for your health. Diabetic friendly baking involves using alternative flours like the ones derived from nuts and whole grains. You can use fruit for sweetening or add lemon extract for a lemony flavor. Being diabetic doesn't mean you can't eat baked foods, or that they will kill you. But if you want to reverse your diabetes, you may have to forego them.

Junk Food – Store Bought
Glycemic index: 65 (Flamin' Hot Cheetos)

Sticking with the no processed foods mantra, you will likely have to eliminate most store-bought snacks and treats. Food that belongs in this category are potato chips, Cheetos, pretzels, Chex Mix, dried fruit, candy, powdered doughnuts, you name it. When it comes to junk food, the I-know-it-when-I-see-it classification works for most people. Not only are they empty calories with very little protein or healthy fat content, but they are also full of sugar and processed chemicals. Snacks are not good for you. Even if the label tells you that it is healthy or doctor's choice or some future bastardization of the language, they aren't healthy. Always check the label for impediments and sugar content. You are bound to see sugar in large quantities, high corn syrup, and a slathering of preservatives and other chemicals. The label might not even have sugar but use an alternative like dextrose instead. If you want to be really careful, don't buy them in the first place.

Bottom line: Make healthier snack decisions. You will learn more about portion control and spacing out your meals in later chapters. I want you to eliminate the word "snack" from your vocabulary. Unless your blood glucose falls way below your target range, there is no reason to eat in between major meals. Doing so will only make it harder to hit your goals in the long run. If you really must snack, use healthy alternatives to junk food. A good resource for looking up the sugar content of popular snack foods is www.sugarstacks.com.

Instead, reach for some all-natural fruit! None of that dried stuff which comes packed with sugar preservatives. Though fruit contains fructose, it is in trace amounts and nowhere near the amount of fructose you would consume from snack foods. You can readily find healthy diabetic snack foods online. Some of my favorites include organic, non-sweetened raisins, organic peanut butter on celery sticks or apples, and all kinds of nuts. Raw, unsalted nuts are a good source of fat and are excellent for snacking. You can find raw nuts for sale in bulk at www.nuts.com

Fast Food and sugary drinks
Glycemic Index: 63 (Coca-cola) –
Glycemic Index: 70 (Big Mac)

foods like the kind you purchase from McDonald's and Taco Bell are a big no-no. While sugar isn't a direct concern from the food, refined carbohydrates are. Some of these meals are high in protein, but that that protein comes at a steep price. You have high sodium and lots of empty calories. These foods aren't outright fattening besides the refined carbs, but they also lack good quality nutrients found in all-natural food. Since these foods are calorie dense, you will hit caloric goals very quickly without any benefit whatsoever.

Soda goes hand-in-hand with many a fast food establishment. Sometimes, these places offer "healthier" alternatives along with their fountain drinks like Powerade and Minute Maid Lemonade but these are also high in sugar. Sucralose raises insulin by up to 20% and it's a similar story for the "natural" sweetener stevia. Both aspartame and stevia raise insulin levels higher than sugar does. Artificial sweeteners have also been linked with heart disease. Though in recent years, the global usage of artificial sweeteners skyrocketed, obesity and diabetes rates haven't gone down. The opposite, in fact, is true.

Bottom Line: In recent years, fast food restaurants have put nutritional information about their products online, and in some cases, on the menu itself. It's a good start, but it doesn't mean that the food is healthy. Consumers can pick and choose how many calories they consume, but these menus aren't showing you glycemic indexes, which is what really matters when it comes to weight loss. The simple solution is to eat homemade meals and that is what I recommend. It will take you more time in preparation, but the time you lose will pay dividends when it comes to managing your diabetes and weight-loss.

There are plenty of other things that you can drink, like unsweetened all natural teas. You will be pleased to discover that there are different varieties of teas besides just black. Coffee is another good option, as long as you don't add sugar or creamer. Always remember to drink plenty of water.

Alcohol
Glycemic Index: It varies

Alcoholic drinks are made from the fermentation of sugars and starches. Species of yeasts eat the sugar and convert it into the alcohol we all familiar with. Alcohol itself is not sugar, but many alcoholic drinks have sugary additives. The glycemic index of beer is contested and certainly varies from type of beer and the brand. Beer and liquor that contain maltose score very high in the glycemic index because maltose is almost pure sugar. Sweetened wine also scores high and should probably be avoided. The thing with beer is that it has theorized effects on the metabolism of other carbohydrates in the body. It is theorized that beer consumption can catalyze or accelerate the absorption of carbohydrates, creating a sharp increase in blood sugar. For this reason, beer is considered a high glycemic food by many health professionals. But this is a little misleading because the carbohydrate content of beer and other alcoholic drinks is too low to derive an adequate GI.

Since alcohol is metabolized in the liver, excess alcohol consumption can directly lead to alcoholic fatty liver disease. The excess consumption of alcohol is associated with an increased risk of type 2 diabetes. Moderate alcohol consumption, however, is associated with a reduced risk in type 2 diabetes for those who are already relatively healthy. Alcohol has been proposed to increase insulin sensitivity and a reduction of insulin sensitivity.

Bottom Line:

The key word here is moderation. Most people who are diabetic can enjoy alcohol if it is in moderation. Up to two glasses of unsweetened red wine a day does not raise insulin or affect insulin sensitivity. Nor is it associated with weight gain. If you do plan on drinking alcohol, never drink it by itself, especially not after breaking a fast. Your blood sugar can drop to dangerous levels if you consume alcohol on an empty stomach. This is especially true for those on the low-carb diet.

Pasta
Glycemic Index: 38 (white Spaghetti)

Most pasta you are familiar with is a type of refined carb. The same applies to noodles which a staple food in many Asian cultures. I can sit here and list all the different types of pasta, but I will spare you the trouble. Pasta come in two varieties: dry pasta and fresh pasta. Dried pasta is typically made in a large factory setting while fresh pasta can be pressed at home with a pasta machine or in the store. Despite being a refined carb, pasta tends to score low on the glycemic index. It gets a bad rap because it is easy to skimp on portion control and eat a whole lot of it. If you keep portions no more than 1 cup in size, blood glucose will not spike. But add to these sauces and a side of garlic bread and the calories shoot up. So does blood glucose.

Bottom Line:

Diabetics tend to have a love-hate relationship with pasta. Some avoid at all costs, and others eat it regularly but feel guilty the whole time. Still, others are able to eat it in moderation and have learned techniques to integrate their love for pasta into their diabetes diet. Since this book is about the low-carb diet, you probably don't want to eat too much of the stuff. Use it as a side dish rather than the main one because you are then more likely to gorge on it. If you must eat pasta, go for the low-carb options. There are whole wheat versions of pretty much every pasta out there. Other varieties are high in protein and fiber. You can lower the portion size and add starchy vegetables like squash to make up for the lost pasta. Finally, you can cook it "al dente" or "to the tooth" rather than overcook it. Well-cooked pasta tends to raise insulin levels more than usual so avoid it. Al dente should be chewy but not mushy to eat.

At the end of the day, white pasta is a refined grain. I personally wouldn't eat it with my diabetes diet plan because most pasta is highly processed.

Rice
Glycemic Index: 93 (Pelde Rice)

Believe it or not, rice is a staple food for half of the world population. It is cheap, easy to farm, and above all, it's pretty tasty. White rice, in particular, is considered a refined grain. Observant readers will make the connection between refinement and the color white. Sound dieting advice for any diabetic is to avoid eating anything that is white. This is true for flour, sugar, pasta, and of course, rice. Certain varieties of rice like Pelde rice score abysmally high on the glycemic index.

Other white rice has a lower glycemic index like 53 for Basmati rice. The different values in blood glucose response have been attributed to the presence of a certain starch called amylose. Rice, on average, contains 20% amylose but may be higher or lower based on the variety. Research has shown that rice that is high in amylose scores lower on the glycemic index and rice that has less amylose (some varieties have none) score higher.

As with other forms of grains, the brown whole variety is healthier for you. Brown rice has smaller glycemic indexes than the white version of the same variety. Brown rice is also richer in fiber, minerals, and antioxidants. Making the switch from brown rice has proven to be good for weight loss and lowering cardiovascular disease risk.

Bottom Line: Avoid eating white rice at all costs. Its high glycemic load is not worth the risk of eating it. If you do eat rice, make sure you know what variety it is and look up its GI online. Always shoot for the low ones. Substitute white rice with brown. So-called "weight lost friendly" rice derived foods like rice cakes and puffed rice cereals also have a high GI and should be avoided.

Quinoa
Glycemic Index: 53

Many lump quinoa along with rice, but it is actually an edible seed from a plant. It may serve as a good substitute for rice because of its relatively low glycemic index. It comes in different varieties of red, white, and black. The seed is high in fiber, protein, and vitamins. It also contains a healthy dosage of antioxidants. Though technically a seed, many consider Quinoa to be a whole grain. Since it has grain like properties, it has been used to create low-carb versions of bread, pasta, and even polenta.

Bottom Line: Quinoa is considered a low-GI food and is preferable to rice. It has the highest protein content of any grain (even though it's a seed) plus fiber. Quinoa is a good choice for your carbohydrate requirements. The only complaint I have with it and what others commonly nag about is that it has a bland taste. If that is an issue for you, considering using lime juice or adding flavorful veggies to make a salad.

Beans
Glycemic Index: 33 (pinto bean)

Beans are a type of legume that is high in protein, vitamins, and minerals. They are a staple food for many regions of central and southern America including Mexico but only make up a fraction of the American diet. Despite scoring low in the glycemic index, beans tend to be high in carbohydrate content. A single cup of pinto beans contains roughly 91 grams of net carbs. Beans are great for a side dish and should never be used as the main source of protein in a low carb diet. Even just two servings (one cup) of beans goes well over the carb limit on most diets. For this reason, all type of beans is discouraged in the lowest carb-diets. The ketogenic diet generally disallows them, as does Paleo. There is no way you could eat beans for the carbohydrate requirement of the Atkins 40 diet because just one serving goes over the total limit.

Bottom Line: Beans should be avoided on low-carb diets. They have many benefits and a low GI score, but the carb content is high. They can be enjoyed in moderation, though. More forgiving diets like a lenient LCHF or a Banting diet may be able to accommodate them.

Whole Fruits and Berries
Glycemic Index: 40 (Blue Berry)
Glycemic Index: 38 (Apples)

Fruits are a type of carbohydrate that is high in fructose. Most fruits score low on the glycemic index with the exception of a select few. Additionally, a large portion of a fruit's weight comes in the form of water. Their water content makes you feel fuller after eating. Berries are also low-GI foods and are high in antioxidants. Blueberries are a keto favorite. Berries tend to have lower carbohydrate counts than fruits and so should be preferred. Fruits should be eaten in moderation because of their fructose and carbohydrate content.

Bottom Line: While there is some wiggle room for berries in low-carb diets, there is less room for fruits. You definitely don't want to eat more than one serving of fruit a day (even that makes up a good portion of carbs). Instead, consider eating smaller amounts of fruits. Instead of eating a whole apple which is around 18 grams of net carb, consider cutting it in half.

Starchy Vegetables
Glycemic index: 63 (Sweet potatoes)

A starch is a type of polysaccharide (sugar) contained in certain vegetables like potatoes, corn, chickpeas, pumpkin, and zucchini to name a few. You will want to avoid most of these on a low-carb diet because they tend to have high carb counts with a few exceptions. Sweet potatoes are lower in carbs than white potatoes, but both are still high. Zucchini, on the other hand, is very low in carbohydrates and can be enjoyed alongside meals.

Bottom Line: Potatoes make up a big portion of the American diet, but they are too carby for many low-carb diets. You shouldn't be eating them. Other starchy vegetables that are low in carbs are good alternatives. Squashes tend to be a good bet.

Non-Starchy Vegetables
Glycemic Index: 10 (Broccoli)

Non-starchy vegetables are like the holy grail of low-carb diets. You will get most of your carbohydrate needs from these foods. They have low GI scores across the board and are a good source of vitamins and minerals. Vegetables in this group include broccoli, peppers, cabbage, lettuce, onion, mushroom, tomato, eggplant, and cauliflower. You can enjoy these foods raw or cooked depending on the dish you are making and your personal taste.

Bottom line: There is little else to say. You need to incorporate non-starchy vegetables into your low-carb diet. The Atkins 40 refers to them as the "foundational vegetables" that make up the diet. And for good reason too.

Proteins

It is a common belief that only carbohydrates raise insulin. In fact, all three of the macronutrients have the potential to raise insulin. Protein doesn't affect blood glucose like a carbohydrate, instead, it gets broken down into amino acids for muscle repair and the creation of new tissues. Ingesting proteins also result in another process. The stomach releases hormones called incretins which release insulin to help bring down blood glucose. Since every food has an insulin response, it is easy to see why people get so caught up with counting calories. The more you eat the more insulin your body produces. The more insulin your body produces, the fatter your body stores, and ultimately, you gain weight. However, it is insulin, not excess calories, that contributes the most to gaining weight. The incretin effect is behind the failure of many high protein diets for weight loss.

Protein sources have always been lauded for their health benefits. Their consumption promotes muscle growth and good bone health. They are especially popular among low-carb dieters who put a premium on the number of calories derived from protein sources. But if you are diabetic, you don't want to splurge on eating meats. Since proteins can and do raise insulin levels, you are going to want to put a limit on how much you eat. Of course, you should still eat more protein than carbohydrates. Carbohydrates raise insulin levels much greater than the release of incretins. The two main sources of protein in non-vegan diets come in the form of meat and dairy. Dairy scores pretty low on the glycemic index at around 15-30 but scores moderately on the insulin index. That is, dairy consumption has a strong effect on raising insulin levels. That still doesn't mean you should give it up altogether. The relationship between protein and insulin is a complicated one.

Besides raising insulin, incretins have several other functions. One of these is to create the feeling of satiety or feeling full. We all know that food is broken down by chewing and saliva then goes down the esophagus and into the stomach where stomach acids further help digest the food. Incretins control the amount of time the stomach takes to absorb food before releasing it into the intestines. This essentially stops you from craving additional food until your stomach is emptied again. Imagine consuming 400 calories of steak versus 400 calories of ice cream. Ice cream digests fast meanwhile the steak stays in your stomach for longer. It's almost as if you can feel the steak just sitting there slowly digesting. Curiously enough, the satiety effect promotes weight-loss because you are less prone to binge eating. Doubtless, you have probably been to one of those all-you-can-eat style buffets sometime in your life. You arrive there with an empty stomach and consume a variety of foods. Let's say that you load your plate with chicken wings, pork cutlets, and shrimp. For your next round, you get the fried shrimp, teriyaki chicken, and some tasty cuts of flank steak. By the time you get to your third plate, you begin to slow down. Even though it is all you can eat, your full stomach prevents you from gaming the system and eating anymore.

There is a phenomenon people often talk about called the "second stomach". Despite being full from high-protein meals, people can still "make room" for dessert if it is high in sugar and refined carbohydrates. This has less to do with hunger and all to do with pleasure eating. Following a low-carb diet will prevent you from developing the second stomach mentality.

Incretins then have two opposing effects. They raise insulin, which causes weight gain, and they promote satiety, which caused weight loss. Do these two effects cancel each other out? There is a reason to believe so, but like most things discussed in this book, it's complicated. For one, not all types of protein have the same incretin response. Dairy raises insulin levels significantly, but most people can't eat several portions of dairy in one sitting. A glass of milk or piece of cheese is the preferred portion sizes. You don't see people wolfing down gallons of milk unless they are on some crazed bodybuilder diet.

I will discuss the main sources of protein in our diets and how you should go about integrating them into your low-carb routine.

Beef
Insulin Index: 51 ± 12

Red meat is an excellent option for getting in your daily protein needs. If you want to target both protein and fat at the same time, go for fatty cuts of meat. Popular cuts of meat include chuck, sirloin, ribeye, flank, and skirt. You can also buy ground beef for making your own burgers. Ground beef comes in different varieties varying on fat content. If you are trying to reach ketoses faster, it is recommended to go with the fatty kind. If you have heart concerns, you may wish to limit consumption of red meat. It is very important to keep up with the portion control when decorating your plate with food. Beef is good and has virtually no limit for diabetics, but you still shouldn't gorge on it. Of course, since you are following a low-carb diet that is mostly high in fat, you won't be eating too much meat. The insulin index is based on the insulin response of pure white bread which averages out about 100. In this case, beef has a score of 51 give or take 12. This makes it a mid-range insulin-secreting food. You are going to want to avoid eating cured meats like sausages, hot dogs, and bacon because they tend to be highly processed. If possible, purchase all your meat from a local butcher.

Bottom Line: The many cuts of beef make it a versatile food. You don't have to eat the same type of cut over and over again. Additionally, the fat content in beef is high relative to the other sources of protein listed below. Beef goes really well with stir fry recipes that you can load up with non-starchy vegetables like peppers and onion.

Poultry
Insulin Index: 19 (Chicken pan-fried w/ skin

For those who do not like beef or wish to get protein from elsewhere, poultry is an excellent option. It has inherently less fat than beef, but some fatty cuts are available like chicken thighs. Chicken breasts are incredibly lean. You can buy a whole chicken rather cheaply and you can even make a delicious bone broth out of it. Poultry has an insulin index of 19, which is significantly lower than that of beef. You are going to want to avoid seasonings and dips such as barbecue and honey. This goes for all types of meat, not just poultry. Eat the food cooked with as little seasoning as possible. Avoid all breaded chicken. Pan frying is okay, but you probably want to skip on the Churches chicken deal or the KFC bucket. The breaded chicken comes with added carbs that you do not want. As always, avoid processed deli meats. No more turkey ham sandwiches!

Bottom Line: Poultry may be a better option than meat for many people. It tends to be cheaper and has less fat. A common complaint with poultry is that it is bland or tasteless. You will want to resist the urge to use overly indulgent seasoning sauces. Spices are generally okay.

Eggs
Insulin Index: 31 ± 6

Eggs are one of the best breakfasts a diabetic can have. High in essential proteins, potassium, and other nutrients, the egg is a powerhouse. It is debatable whether the cholesterol content of eggs is bad for you or not. In recent years, eggs have been lauded as healthy even with their cholesterol content. They also have a relatively low insulin index. You can eat them scrambled, in omelets, hardboiled, or even raw. You can add them to your other meals. A steak topped with a fresh egg is a delicious dinner or lunch. Most of the egg's nutrients come from the yolk, so make sure you eat them raw. Beware that eggs have at least one gram of net carbs, and should be counted accordingly

Bottom Line: You really can't go wrong with eggs whether you are doing the ketogenic diet or a more moderate low-carb one. If you suffer from high cholesterol, eggs might not be the best option for you. You should go over these concerns with your doctor.

Fish
Insulin Index: 43 (white fish fillet)

Fish is also highly recommended for diabetics. Most types of white fish (tilapia, trout, cod) are relatively inexpensive but can be pricey for some. Tilapia tends to be leaner while salmon and trout are high in omega-3 fatty acids. The omega-3 make them an excellent choice of healthy fat. Fish fillets are generally easy to prepare. Thin cuts of tilapia and salmon can easily be sautéed on a stove top using a non-stick pan. If you prefer grilling fish, cod is really good. Counting calories is simplified with shrimps as they have straightforward portions, but they are high in cholesterol. Canned tuna has a long shelf live and is cheap. Go for tuna in oil if you want to increase fat content or use water for a leaner choice. Unfortunately, you are going to want to avoid eating sushi. Though marketed as "raw" fish, the rice and seaweed wrap make it high in carbohydrates. If you are a big fan of the raw fish, there are leaner options available that don't contain rice like sashimi.

Bottom Line: Include fish in your diet to create a varied protein intake. As always, avoid using added seasonings and sugars. Squirting a few lemons on top of white fish is usually good enough for the taste. Do not bread your fish, and stay away from breaded fish products like fish fingers and patties.

Dairy
Insulin Index: 39 ± 3

Dairy is a protein source that also contains carbs. One serving of whole milk is about one cup and contains some 15 net carbs. Dairy isn't really fattening if eating in moderation. Cheeses, plain yogurt, and butter are also filling. Even small portions of these foods will keep you satisfied. Dairy is inherently a heavy food, meaning that you are less likely to gorge on it. As long as dairy fits your macros, you can eat it liberally. You don't have to worry about 2% of low-fat milk either. You can eat those other types, but the difference in your diet will be negligible. Note that you will have to count the carbohydrates in whatever dairy you chose. In extremely low-carb diets like keto, dairy can reach your carb requirements quickly. Also, we aren't talking about sugary dairy products like ice-cream and low-fat yogurt. Keep your sources as whole and unprocessed as possible.

Whey Protein, Shakes, Meal Replacements
Insulin Index: Varies

Whey protein is a by-product of the dairy product creation process, mostly from cheeses. Bodybuilders use it in a powdered form with water or milk to create shakes. While these sources are high in protein, they are highly processed. In the consumer sphere, you have products like Ensure and Boost. All of these products including most whey powders are extremely high in carbohydrates. A single serving of Ensure can net as many as 36 carbs. These products were designed to get extra protein in people who don't get enough of it in their diets. Or for "body-builders" who need an extra protein source. Boost and Ensure are sometimes prescribed to patients with wasting diseases that have lost a significant portion of fat and muscle stores. In other words, they are people looking to gain weight rather than lose it. Most people on the low-carb diet can get all of their protein needs from the above meats and there is no need to go this route. I highly discourage the use of any of these whey and chemical concoctions.

Fats

The war against dietary fat started around the 1950s with the rise of nutritionism in the United States. Foods were considered harmful or good based solely on nutritional values. If avocados had the same amount of fat in them than butter, then avocados are no better than butter. Today, avocados are considered a super food by many in the industry. All fats were treated the same including saturated, polyunsaturated, and unsaturated fat. Fat was hardly thought of being beneficial, it was more like a risk appetite that everyone had to tolerate with their choice of foods that contained it. Omega 6 fats, for example, are a polyunsaturated fatty acid used in vegetable oils. Omega 6 has inflammatory properties that can worsen cardio-vascular conditions. Their appearance in our diet only started without the ability to process tons of vegetables at once. Corn is not rich in oil normally. But if you crush a whole bunch of them, you get some semblance of oil. In contrast, omega 3 fats occur naturally in seeds, nuts, and oily fish. Omega 3 has anti-inflammatory properties and can lower the risk of thrombosis. Native populations who live near the ice caps have a diet high in omega 3 fats from fish and whale blubber, yet their cardiovascular health is stellar. A high omega 6 to omega

3 fatty acid ratio in the body causes inflammation. Most Americans consume more omega 6 and not enough omega 3. The war against butter resulted in the creation of margarine, a far deadlier food. Margarine was originally made using trans fats. Both margarine and vegetable oils are as synthetic a food as you can get. The point here is that most fats you find in an unprocessed natural state are safe to eat. Of the three macronutrients, fats are least likely to stimulate insulin.

Olive and Coconut Oil
Insulin Index: 3 (Olive Oil)

Olive oil has long been recognized for its health properties. Even in ancient times, olives have been cultivated for their oil. The process for making other vegetable oils is more than just a matter of crushing. It involves bleaching the vegetable, adding chemicals, and then extracting the resulting "oil". In contrast, olive oil is a matter of crushing the olive into a paste and then extracting the oil using a press. It is very mechanically involved, but no more than what the average ancient civilization in 4500 BC could achieve. This oil is natural and requires zero chemicals. Virgin olive oils mean that they were created using just the mechanical process described above. Other varieties may be refined, and contain added chemicals. Extra-virgin means that the oil is still refined but has an extra standard of quality and taste. The health benefits of olive oil are astounding. It has anti-inflammatory properties, large amounts of anti-oxidants help lower cholesterol and blood pressure, and decreases blood clotting. In order words, olive oil helps treat cardiovascular disease.

Coconut oil is full of medium-chain triglycerides (MCT). These fatty acids are shorter than other varieties of bad fats and can reduce the risk of heart disease. MCT's go straight to the liver where they are used as energy or become ketones. Consequently, coconut oil increases your metabolism and burns more fat. High in saturated fats, coconut oil furthermore increases good cholesterol called HDL.

Bottom Line: You need to increase your intake of these oils. At the very least, get more olive oil. While you increase intake of good oils, you want to decrease or eliminate the intake of bad oils. Vegetable oils and corn oils should be removed. You can cook virtually anything with olive and coconut oil. A quick breakfast is some sautéed non-starchy vegetables in olive oil. You can also make olive oil into various dips and sauces. Anywhere you would normally use butter, you can also use olive oil.

Butter and beef tallow
Insulin Index: 2 (butter)

Butter is a dairy product that is completely made up of fat. It is high in saturated fats that raise HDL or good cholesterol. Butter also contains the fatty acid butyrate which is anti-inflammatory and has powerful effects on the digestive system. Not to mention that butter is completely delicious. It is easily eaten along carby foods like bread and pancakes, so you will have to think about other ways to include it in your diet. The simple solution is to add it to every meal during the cooking process.

Beef tallow is a kind of butter, but it is made out of beef or mutton fat. It is often sold in blocks or as a cream in a jar. It can even be used as an ingredient in bars of soap. The consistency is a cross between coconut oil and butter. You can use it for any type of cooking that requires high heat such as sautéing, stir-frying, and grilling.

Bottom Line: Both butter and beef tallow are derived from pure, all-natural sources. Beef tallow comes straight from animal fat and butter is made from milk cream. Either one of these choices is legions better than margarine. If you are still eating that plastic margarine stuff, now is the time to throw it out. While you might have to get a little inventive for eating these in your low-carb diet, the benefits make up for it.

Nuts
Insulin Index: 5 (walnuts)

Nuts are prominently featured in Mediterranean style diets, which are considered one of the healthiest out there for weight loss. Nuts are both low in carbohydrates and high in natural fats. Some nuts have higher carbohydrate content than others and may need to be factored in toward your carbohydrate counts. Foods derived from nuts like all-natural peanut butter are good ways to enjoy nuts. If you are going this route, you need to find a peanut butter that has no sugar and little to no carbs.

Avocado
Insulin Index: 4

Avocados are a strange, wondrous freak of nature. Most fruits are high in carbohydrates and fructose, but not avocados. Instead, they are high in fats. They are highly nutritious, with a long list of vitamins that include potassium, vitamin C, vitamin E, vitamin B5, and vitamin B6. Avocados are high fiber, meaning that net carbs are very low. It is the perfect diabetic food on a low-carb diet. People mostly associate potassium with bananas, but avocados can contain more. Since they are less carby, avocados give you an alternative option for potassium needs. Potassium can help reduce blood pressure.

Chapter 4: Effective Low Carb Diet with Healthy Habits

By now, you have heard about all of the benefits of the low carb diet. You should have a good idea of what kinds of low-carb diets are out there and which one you'd like to use for your diabetes management. You should also have an idea of what type of foods you can have and how your meals will look. A low-carb diet is only half of the battle of managing diabetes. But don't feel discouraged, as this is a step in the right direction. I figure that finding diabetic recipes is easy enough online, so I won't include any here. I will talk about the dreaded exercise, as well as using intermittent fasting as another tool in your arsenal against diabetes. I can already picture some of you rolling your eyes at the mere mention of the word fasting. It's funny because you already fast on a daily basis every time you go to sleep. Fasting is practiced all over the world by distinct cultures and religions. If the Hindus, Buddhists, and Muslim populations can do it, so can you. If well over a quarter of the world population can fast, then so can you.

Healthy Habit # 1 Beware of the big breakfast

Ever since we are in grade school, we are pounded with the idea that a healthy, full breakfast is the key to optimal nutrition. We hear such expressions like "breakfast is the most important meal of the day". The truth is, breakfast is optional. For too many people use breakfast as an excuse to gorge themselves with food first thing in the morning. And what kind of things do we eat in the morning? We have a plethora of sugary breakfast cereal, sweet bread, pancakes, doughnuts, bagels, English muffins, and sugary concoctions from your local Starbucks. Notice that all of these foods are either high in sugar or refined carbohydrates. Not the ideal way to start your day by any means. Yet, the food companies that advertise these products benefit from pushing the "most important meal of the day" agenda.

The notion that a single meal is the most important is preposterous. There is no such thing. All meals are equally important, especially when it comes to regulating your blood sugar. A simple protocol you can follow for breakfast is to ask yourself two questions. One, are you hungry? If you are not hungry, then don't eat. It is as simple as that. Too often, we assume that breakfast is the only meal we will have until later, so we tend to eat preemptively even if we aren't all that hungry. Breaking a fast at lunchtime has little differences from breaking a fast at 8 am. The second question you should ask yourself is how is my blood sugar? If you wake up and notice that it is a little on the low side, you should definitely eat something to get it back to your prescribed range.

Many diabetics have breakfast every day as part of their dieting plan. That is perfectly okay as long as you keep your calories light. The real problem belongs to the "full" or "big" breakfast that is often advertised as healthy. Using the low-carb diet you shouldn't be eating doughnuts, sweet bread, most breakfast cereals, or bagels. A healthy light breakfast may consist of a cup of coffee, an omelet, and a side of berries. Don't overdo it with too many eggs or dairy. No large "English" style breakfast or Grand Slams from Denny's.

Healthy Habit #2 Portion Control

You probably don't need a huge breakfast anyways. Eating too much will cause your blood glucose to shoot up beyond your prescribed range. In fact, putting too much on your plate at any meal is bad for your diabetes. A better option is to control the size of each meal so that your blood sugar goes up in a controlled manner. You will have to learn how to stop binge eating if that is a problem for you. Even if you don't eat a lot at meals, you should still learn how to portion out your food. Since a low-carb diet is often low in processed foods, you will have to learn how to measure your food portions on your own. Say goodbye to neat caloric details on the back of the package. Don't worry, portioning your meals is relatively simple. It only slightly adds to the overall food preparation cost.

The first thing you need to know about is measurements. The good news is that you don't need precise measuring equipment for gauging how much food you are looking at. There are simple rules that can guide you in this pursuit. Having measuring utensils never hurts, but not everyone will have access to them. Below is a general list of tips for gauging the portion of commonly used food.

- One serving of meat is around three ounces, the rough equivalent of a standard deck of playing cards. One ounce is about one-sixteenth of a pound
- Solid dairy (cheese, yogurt, etc.) should be in the form of one ounce per serving. This is equivalent to six standard playing dice.
- One serving of fruit is about the size of a tennis ball.
- One serving of raw leafy greens is one cup. Another way to measure this is by using both hands. However, much produce fits in both your hands is about one cup.
- One serving of cooked greens is a ½ cup, or about what you can carry in a single hand.
- One serving of bread is about one slice.
- One serving of rice or cooked pasta is one-third cup.
- Potato or Corn about ½ cup
- Dry cereal about ¾ cup

- One serving of alcohol is either 12 ounces of beer or six ounces of wine

Food intake should be regulated by your blood glucose levels rather than hunger. At the minimum, you should check blood glucose levels before each major meal. If you consider breakfast, lunch, and dinner as the major meals, then that is three times you will check. Sometimes, it is recommended that diabetics eat more frequent, smaller meals to better regulate blood glucose. More frequent meals though cause insulin levels to rise and if there isn't enough time in between them, then insulin levels won't go down as normal. In any case, speak with your doctor before changing up your meal frequency. If you already eat 3-4 meals a day and that works for you, then it's better to stick to it. If your doctor recommended more meals, then you should comply. Note that meal frequency is directly tied with the oral medications you are taking, including insulin treatments, so it is paramount that you speak with your doctor about this.

Never skimp on fit your portions to your meals. A serving refers to the minimum amount of food used to derive caloric and nutritional content. A portion, on the other hand, refers to the amount of food you will consume in one sitting. If your diabetic diet calls for 3 servings of fruit in one day, you could split those up by eating one apple, orange, or pear with each meal. Or you could eat one apple at breakfast, half a banana for lunch, and the rest of the banana with dinner. A full-size banana is typically two servings of fruit.

The distinction between serving size and portions is extremely important when eating packaged food. Consider the container for a sugary drink (not that you should be drinking it in the first place). Though the label says that a serving is 12 ounces, the bottle may contain 20. A full-size candy bar might have half or even half of half as a single serving. Some of these foods are designed to be eaten all at once, and you imagine what that does to your diet. Read packaging carefully to get the adequate serving size and fit it to your portions for that meal.

Consider using portion plates, measuring cups, and spoons to really streamline the process of counting your portions. Also buy smaller plates, bowls, and cups so that you are less likely to go over your allotted portion size. The rest is really all up to you. If you get hungry between a meal, do not snack because it will go over your allotted portions. If after finishing a meal you go for seconds or thirds, you are also going over your allotted portion size. The simple answer is not to do it. Choose combinations of foods that are naturally filling like quality animal meat at each meal.

Healthy Habit #3 Intermittent Fasting

So, eliminating sugars and refined carbohydrates from the diet limits the rise in blood glucose. Limiting the rise in blood glucose lowers insulin levels. Lowering insulin levels decreases insulin resistance, which in turn also lowers insulin. The lower your insulin levels, the less excess glucose there is, the less glucose is available to be converted into fat. But what happens if you already have large stores of fat? Limiting the creation of new fat through diet is a good step, but sometimes, it needs to get rid of the fat that has accumulated in visceral organs and under the skin. Additionally, fasting breaks the endless insulin-resistance cycle you get from constant insulin spikes. When you fast, you experience zero glucose spikes which only lowers the insulin response. If frequent eating and snacking are bad for insulin levels, then zero eating is the antidote. Since all foods increase insulin, the only way to lower it is by not consuming those foods.

Remember what I said about the basal metabolic rate in previous chapters. Even if you eat fewer calories, the number of calories you burn daily shifts so that you don't starve to death. First glucose stores need to deplete. Once that happens, your body goes into a state of ketosis where fat is broken down into ketone bodies you can use for energy. Ketosis is able to burn fat without you even doing anything. One way to reach ketosis as prescribed by the ketogenic diet is to severely limit consumption of carbohydrates. Another way to achieve ketosis is to simply not eat for extended periods of time. The prime reason why calorie-restrictive diets don't work is that the body is provided with just enough fuel to sustain critical systems. If someone eats 1000 calories from a carb-rich diet, their body says "Oh hey, look energy! It's not what I usually get, so I will make do with what I have" The amount of fat in their system remains the same. The amount of glucose in the blood, though lower, will also remain stable. Bodily functions necessary for life like blood circulation and brain metabolism is slowed just enough to preserve the body. Your body will do all that it can to squeeze out the last drop of glucose it has. This is what we normally refer to as starvation mode, and it is vastly different from ketosis.

Under ketosis, the body says "Uh oh, I'm on empty. I need to break open the old fat storage safe so I can get the energy I need to survive". You have more energy during ketosis than during starvation mode because your body knows it needs the energy to find food. In prehistoric times, this energy was needed to hunt, scavenge, and forage. But you don't have to go to prehistoric extremes to benefit from fasting. You already fast every night for (hopefully) 6 – 8 hours. What's another 8 or 10 hours?

Realistically speaking, you won't reach ketosis by simply not eating for ten hours. The body's response to starvation is complex. It can be summed up in 5 sequential steps

1. **Normal Eating**

This is fairly obvious. You eat something, and the body turns it into energy. Insulin rises to increase blood glucose uptake. Cells that can directly use glucose for energy take what is needed. The muscles, brain, and organ systems are included. Whatever excess glucose remains is directed to the liver where it is stored as glycogen.

2. **Six to 24 hours after eating**

As glucose gets used up, insulin levels fall. Once the muscles, brain, and organ systems are depleted of energy from blood glucose, the glycogen stores inside the liver begin to convert into glucose. Glycogen stores can last up to 24 hours.

3. **Twenty-four hours to two days after eating**

In glycogenesis, non-carbohydrate sources get converted into glucose. These include glycerol and amino acids.

4. **One to three days after eating**

Ketosis. Fat in the form of triglycerides is broken down into three fatty acids. Some structures in the body can directly use this fat for energy but not the brain. Fatty acid further broken down into ketone bodies which power 75% of bodily function.

5. **Five days and beyond**

Five days after the last eating, the body desperately tries to preserve muscle mass by releasing growth hormone. Basal metabolic function is purely powered by fatty acids and ketones. Increased adrenaline secretion prevents metabolism from falling.

It takes at least 24 hours for ketosis to begin after the last meal. The best way to use intermittent fasting is in the form of 24 to 36-hour fasts twice a week. Once you are in that ketosis face, you can burn fat for free.

If I still haven't convinced you that fasting is desirable, consider the many different diets that are out there. Dieting is complex, expensive, and time-consuming. Meal prep takes up time and effort. Healthy foods that are organic or free-range are prohibitively expensive for some. With fasting, you don't need to spend time or money. It simply works without you having to do anything.

How to successfully fast

The rules for fasting are simple. You are allowed to drink non-caloric fluids, take medications, and use a multivitamin. All forms of calorie consumption are not allowed until the fast is over. You are probably wondering what happens with your blood sugar. Not eating for extending periods of time will cause hypoglycemic conditions, yes. But not for long. Ketosis kicks in, and you receive a boost in energy. If you are taking medication, you must speak with your doctor before trying out a fasting regimen. This is non-negotiable. The medication that you take while on the fast may result in hypoglycemia. If this happens and you are required to consume sugar to get blood glucose back up, you will effectively break the fast. Since you won't be eating anything, blood sugar shouldn't spike. If it does go above your targeted range, you will have to medicate accordingly.

Blood glucose may spike in the morning. This is sometimes called the "dawn phenomenon". Normally, the body's circadian rhythm readies itself for the coming day. Your body secretes adrenaline, cortisol, and several other hormones to give you a wake-up kick. In diabetics, the fatty liver desperately wants to get rid of its glycogen stores, so it releases glucose into the bloodstream. This reaction is expected and is evidence that the body is starting its sugar detox. If you aren't eating anything, where else would the glucose come from? From inside your body of course. You should expect the dawn phenomena right after your first fast, but it can also occur later. Your body will get used to it the more you practice fasting. If blood sugar is outside your target range, medicate accordingly.

Start your fast by checking your blood glucose level and drinking at least 8 ounces of water. If you get bored of just plain water, you can add lime juice or cut up slices of oranges and other citruses in a large pitcher to diffuse taste. All sorts of black and green teas are permitted if they are zero calories. Coffee caffeinated or decaffeinated is also allowed but no sweeteners whatsoever. A little bit of milk or creamer is okay despite having some calories. For longer fasts, you can use homemade bone broth made from beef, pork, or chicken bones. These broths will help keep sodium levels up. When the fast is over, make sure to break it with a small meal. Eating too much may upset your stomach or give you a gnarly headache.

You will feel spells of hunger. The best way to deal with them is to take plenty of antioxidants found in coffee and green tea. Try to keep yourself busy throughout the day as an occupied mind is able to ignore hunger signals. Other symptoms include dizziness, muscle cramps, and headaches. Dizziness is primarily due to dehydration, so drink plenty of water. Both muscle cramps and headaches may be due to low sodium intake. Heat up bone breath with sea salt crystals, take a magnesium pill, or try a relaxing Epson salt bath. At first, you will experience lethargy, but once ketosis kicks in, you should feel more energized. If the lethargy is persistent, it is time to check your blood sugar levels.

Diabetics will need close monitoring from a health professional. If you try to fast, your doctor needs to know when you are doing it and for how long. They should know your glucose levels as well. A doctor's approval is also recommended because they have a complete list of the medications you are on. Some medications for blood pressure can cause lightheadedness. If medications need to be taken with foods, you can try taking them with a small serving of leafy greens. Insulin medications will bring your blood sugars down. In cases of hypoglycemia, you need to take sugar or glucose tablets to get levels to your normal range. If you feel any persistent symptoms of a headache, low energy, diarrhea, or vomiting, stop the fast immediately and seek medical assistance.

If you decide to exercise while fasting, keep your routine light. Do not exercise if your blood sugars are too high or too low.

There is no magic formula that will make fasting work for you. You will need to experiment with the frequency and duration of fasts. A common light fast used by many consists of 8 hours of sleep and another 8 hours of waking fast. This is a grand total of 16 hours, with an 8-hour window for eating. More intense fast include 24 hour and 36-hour fasts. For the 24-hour fast, you eat dinner the first day and don't eat until dinner the following day. Still, there have been cases of morbidly obese diabetics fasting for several weeks or even months at a time for good weight-loss results. A good place to start is with 16-hour fasts. You can do them every other day, three times a week, or on every weekday. Or you can spread two 24 or 36-hour fasts into your week. Monday starts with a 36 hour fast, followed by another on Wednesday or Thursday. You will need to do the necessary "bookwork" to track weight-loss and blood-sugar levels to see what regimen works best for you.

Healthy Habit # 4 Get Moving

While the total amount of calories burned from moderate exercise pale in comparison to the basal metabolic rate, these small increments of caloric energy are enough to create long-term weight loss. Not only that, but exercise benefits you in several different ways. You don't have to run marathons or lift 100 pounds over your head to reap these benefits. As little as 30 minutes of aerobic exercise 4 to 7 days a weak may be all the exercise that you need. Of course, you can always add intensity or frequency if you wish to.

The obvious benefit is that it gets out of the couch or computer chair. These environments entice you to eat more. When we prepare a meal, our first inclination is to get beside a screen so that you can watch something while eating. This is a bad habit that needs to be stopped. It causes you to gulp your food down rather than thoroughly chew it, and it conditions your brain to associate screen watching with eating. If you remove yourself from those environments even if just for a little, you are fighting the urge to eat.

Exercise gets the blood pumping and heart rate going. Both of these provide long-term benefits for cardiovascular disease. Even if you don't go into exercise for the weight loss, these two benefits alone are why you should be exercising. Remember that diabetics have an increased risk of heart attack and stroke. Exercising regularly at a moderate pace is one of the best things you can do to lower risk. That and quitting smoking.

No matter what age you are, we could all use a little more muscle tone. You use your muscles every day. Big, large muscle groups like the legs and upper body are only used during movement. If you are still for the majority of the day, these muscles aren't getting the proper workout.

Exercising temporarily takes your blood sugar down, which can be helpful a few hours after taking a heavy meal.

The Four Don'ts in Diabetic habits

Diet alone can only get you so far if you have otherwise bad habits. Here is a list of things that you have to rally against with all your willpower. It might be hard at first, but with more practice, you gain the necessary momentum to overcome them.

1. NO SNACKS

The low-carb diets presented in this book are designed to be as satisfying as possible. If you do snack, let it be for the purpose of raising your blood glucose into your target ranges. Do not use snack food if you get hungry in between meals. You are better off resisting that hunger, but if you can't, use low-carb foods that still fit your macros. Do not eat health bars, granola pieces, trail mixes, or chocolate. Dark chocolate is okay in moderation, but you would be doing yourself a favor reaching for an apple or celery sticks instead.

2. NO SUGAR

This is one of the hardest habits to build over time if you are used to eating sugar. For obvious reasons, you can't have sugar in your daily meals. The only exception is on the rare holiday or family celebration but even then, it is preferred you don't.

3. NO EXCUSE FOT NOT EXERCISING

The importance of exercise cannot be overstated. Every time you miss a scheduled workout session, you miss on the health benefits. There are only so many days in a year for you to be missing these appointments with yourself or yoga class. Whenever you slack off, you are letting diabetes get an upper hand. Most of the time, these excuses are lame. "I don't have time to drive to the gym", then walk around your neighborhood. "I can't afford a gym", again, walking is free. The only valid excuse for not exercising is if your blood sugar is too low or too high. But if this is a chronic condition, you will need to talk with your doctor about how you can manage it when it is time to exercise.

4. NO WHITE BREAD

This includes all sorts of bakery products besides loaf bread. No bagels, muffins, cake, or flour tortillas. If you must eat something bready, go for the whole wheat/grain variety. Your best bet is to use a specialty flour like almond and walnut flour.

Chapter 5: Check on Your Progression

Once you have an established low-carb diet and exercise routine, you are all set on your journey to managing diabetes. I hesitate to use the word "cure" because that has yet to be seen in the literature and in personal anecdotes from those who suffer from diabetes. The symptoms of diabetes can be controlled through medication. Through the right diet and exercise, the underlying mechanisms of the disease can be mitigated. But what happens as soon as you stop paying attention to your diet? What happens if you make good progress and you decide to start eating a doughnut every morning as a reward? You probably already know the answer. Blood sugar shoots up, insulin follows, and suddenly, you are diabetic again. Of course, it is a little more complex than this. The more you practice dieting and consuming low-carbohydrate food, the better your body becomes at regulating blood sugar. For many, reaching a comfortable spot between managing the disease, lifestyle, and symptoms is good enough as a cure. I hope you are one of those people.

The obvious markers to record on your journey to managing diabetes are weight and fasting blood glucose. You can also record your hemoglobin A1C score every time your doctor tests you for it. The ultimate goal for most diabetics is to achieve management of the disease without the need for medications. This much is true for type 2 diabetics, but not for those who suffer from type 1. You will still need insulin medications if you have type 1. The type 2 diabetic, however, can enjoy a higher insulin sensitivity using a low-carb diet, regular fasting, and a healthy lifestyle.

Starting a food diary

A food diary doesn't have to be as complex as it sounds. All you need is introductory knowledge of a spreadsheet program like Microsoft Excel or Google Sheets. You can also use old-fashioned paper, but you miss out on the added functionality of spreadsheets. Another option is to use a third-party application on your personal device to track daily meals and blood glucose. Using the spreadsheet option gives you the most control, in my opinion. Keeping a food diary can be hard work for some. The simplest method is to track what you eat in terms of servings and food, along with blood glucose levels two hours after finishing the meal. Its okay if you miss a few entries here and there, the point is to be able to account for your progress.

One column should be dedicated to the date. Next, create a column for each major meal you are scheduled to eat. The simplest is to use breakfast, lunch, and dinner or breakfast, brunch, lunch, then dinner if you do four meals. Beside each of these columns should be another column for recording blood glucose two hours after your meal. If you are more sophisticated, you can track down your macros and calories as well.

As you reach your weight goals, search for places that you can modify your diet. If you are severely overweight or obese, you will directly benefit from a keto diet. But once your weight starts to drop to normal levels, you may consider increasing carb intake. If you like carby food, this will be a form of reward.

The truth is that low-carb diets are difficult to maintain. It is effective at losing weight but it comes at a cost.

Have regular weigh-ins

Don't wait to go to the doctor's office or clinic to be surprised by your weight. Along with blood glucose, you should regularly be tracking your weight. You can either eyeball this or keep a simple notepad. You can also use a spreadsheet. A favorite for me is using a calendar app and writing down my weight on each day. The best time to weigh yourself is in the morning. Besides weight, you might want to track body-fat percentage (BFP) and body-mass index (BMI). As you may or may not know, obesity is classified using BMI.

The easiest way to calculate BFP is to use an online tool like the one at https://www.active.com/fitness/calculators/bodyfat. You will also need to know how to use a measuring tape. You simply input your body measurements, indicate whether you are male or female, and then receive the score. Note that this tool only estimates your BFP using your BMI. Other methods include using body fat calipers to measure skinfolds at key places in the body. The most precise way to get BFP is through sophisticated lab tests. Ask your doctor about these tests if you are interested.

Calculating your BMI is easier. You can use an online calculator, but I will just give you the formula. Since BMI is measured in kilograms, you must first convert your weight from pounds. Alternatively, you can use the formula of mass in pounds divided by height in inches squared multiplied by 703.

You can break down BMI into various categories between genders. There's everything from underweight to extremely underweight and several classes of obesity. In general, though, the normal range is from 18.5 to 3. From 23 to 25, you are considered overweight and at risk of obesity. From 25 to 30, you are considered moderately obese. A BMI above 30 means that you are severely obese.

Track Exercise

I also encourage you to keep a planner or spreadsheet for your workout routines. Depending on the type of exercise, you can track the duration and how much calories you burned. Over time, you can move the same distance in less time by speeding up your pace or breaking into a jog. The most important thing is that you track the date. At the end of the year or month, you can directly see how many days you workout and which days you were supposed to work out but missed. If you use a spreadsheet, you can color code columns to indicate a job well done or a missed day. The more greens you see, the more motivated you are to work out. If you see red, meaning that you missed that workout, you might be motivated to not miss the next one.

It is important to reward your good efforts. Every once in a while, you can take a diabetic friendly dessert. Make sure that sugar is low, and that there are no refined carbs though. You can reward yourself in other ways besides foods. Consider a bath bomb, massage, or Epson salts bath. If you like video games, give yourself some extra gaming sessions.

The cure to diabetes – a multifaceted approach

When oncologists treat cancer, they don't use a single medication. They use "combination therapy" that may include surgery, chemotherapy, and radiotherapy. Even with chemotherapy, doctors prescribe multiple cytotoxic agents rather than just one. Diabetes is no different. Rest assured that your battle with diabetes will be waged on multiple fronts. The diet is the most important, but diet alone will not save you. Medications are important as well, but all they do is control symptoms rather than treat them. A healthy lifestyle is at the core of diabetes management, which includes a healthy diet and adequate exercise. The closest thing we have to a cure for a diabetes is controlling the disease so that your blood glucose is in a permanent state of good levels. Neither too high nor too low. Though achieving those levels is not to say that diabetes is gone for good. If you suddenly go back to eating sugary refined foods, your diabetic problems may very well come back. A low-carb diet, as well as fasting, is an adequate treatment to increase insulin sensitivity, but it can be lost if you don't stick with the diet. Over time, you can increase your carbohydrate intake if they come from whole, nutritious sources.

Remember that diabetes is not a death sentence. Neither is it a recommendation for changing your lifestyle. You need to change your lifestyle or else. If you let diabetes kill you, it will kill you. And it will be painful and miserable for both you and your family. Of all the ways you can go, kidney failure is one of the most dehumanizing. You can live all your life with type 2 diabetes and still have a normal life expectancy as long as you do change your lifestyle to fit it. It's a little crude, but you can think of diabetes as a lifelong friend that is always there watching what you eat. The good thing is that the diabetic lifestyle described in this book is still a healthy one.

Your fight towards conquering diabetics is not yours alone. Your doctor will be there every step as well as your family and support system. I'm telling you right now, if you don't have any diabetic friends, go out and find them. Join online message boards and forums, go to meetups, do what you have to do and find these people. Having someone in your life that shares your condition, your worries, and your triumphs will give you the strength and courage that you need on bad days. And those bad days will happen. You just need to be prepared to meet them. Making a significant change to your lifestyle is not easy.

You need to include your family and support system with you in the fight. Let them know about your goals and notify them about your dietary requirements. They will have to comply with your lifestyle, no matter what. They need to know what you can and cannot eat. Like that one vegan friend, they should be able to respect your dietary decisions. If they can't, or if they refuse to acknowledge all the work that you are doing, I recommend distancing yourself from those people or cutting them off completely. You are going to need all the help on your fight.

And it is doable. There is no shortage of success stories using the low-carb method online and in real life. People have lost astounding amounts of weight by making the switch. You also have the secret weapon of fasting in your arsenal. Among the morbidly obese with diabetes, it is becoming increasingly common to prescribe bariatric surgery as the first line of defense. This surgery effectively makes your stomach the size of a walnut so that calories are incapable of being absorbed. This miraculous surgery is able to control blood sugar levels to non-diabetic levels in a matter of weeks. But you don't have to go to these extremes to have the same results. Bariatric surgery is basically forced fasting until the stomach grows back. The low-carb diet and the right fasting routine can mimic the same effects of the surgery and at a fraction of the cost and risk.

Conclusion

Well, you finally made it to the end of Diabetes Diet: The One Guide to Prevent and Reverse Diabetes

. It is my dearest hope that you gained some useful insights from the information I presented here. If you suffer from diabetes, keep at it. I promise that you can learn to coexist with the condition. It takes some work as I have said countless times in this book, but it is completely possible. Difficult, but reachable goals are one of the best a human being can have.

From here, I encourage you to look up free meal plans online. These are pretty easy to find, all you have to do is look up "low-carb meal plan" or "keto meal plan". There is an endless amount of online communities that are happy to help you along your journey. Stop by the subreddits on Keto and low-carb and I promise you will meet some fellow diabetics there. While these forums aren't diabetic specific, you will be provided with tons of information. If you have a question, feel free to make your own post.

But before you take this into serious consideration, talk to your doctor first. They will be there to guide you and bounce back ideas for your treatment. If you really want to try low-carb, then your doctor will have to put up with it. Heck, you can even find a new one. The low-carb diet is at the heart of an all-natural movement that is out to flush processed food out. We should eat as close to nature as possible. I hope that you too agree.

Lastly, if you enjoyed this book I ask that you please take the time to review it on Audible.com. Your honest feedback would be greatly appreciated.

As always, good luck in your fight against this disease.

Thank you

Now, I would like to share with you a free sneak peek to another one of my books that I think you will really enjoy. The book is called "Self Compassion: The Mindful Path to Understand your Emotions" by Kirstin Germer, Christopher Neff and it's A Practical Guide to Learn the Proven Power of Self-Acceptance, Self-Criticism, Self-Awareness and Mindfulness. You will also learn how to be Kind to Yourself and Move On.

Enjoy!

Introduction

Fostering a sense of self-compassion and self-acceptance can be challenging even for a healthy and well-rounded adult. Despite how important these two characteristics are, very few people are taught about how to utilize them in their personal lives. Instead, we are often taught to be hard on ourselves, push ourselves as far as we can, and demand the maximum results out of our efforts. While challenging yourself to achieve substantial growth is valuable, pushing yourself to the point where it becomes self-sabotaging is not a positive habit to support.

If you truly want to achieve all of the success that you desire in life, you need to have a clear understanding of your mental wellbeing and around how you can support it so that you can improve your chances of succeeding. Without a strong mindset to back them up, most people will fail to achieve their desired level of success because despite having the best of intentions, they will struggle to keep themselves focused and motivated. Through the emotional and mental self-sabotaging behaviors such as having an overly harsh inner critic or trying to push through challenging emotions without acknowledging their purpose or healing them, they will simply burn out and fail to thrive.

As you listen through this book, realize that you are going to be granted every single tool you need to begin developing the skills to become more self-compassionate and self-accepting. From identifying how to feel your emotions and develop a relationship to building a productive mindfulness and self-awareness practice, everything is devoted to helping you motivate yourself in a healthy way. The tools in this book will not encourage or motivate you to become complacent, lose focus, or stop aiming for your dreams with any less intensity than you already have been. Instead, they will support you in having a stronger focus on how you can achieve your goals without compromising your inner sense of wellbeing. As a result, all of the success that you earn in your life will feel far more meaningful and positive.

If self-compassion has been particularly challenging for you until now, or if the concept itself seems foreign, I encourage you to really set the intention to approach this book and the subjects within it with an open mind. You will get the most out of each chapter and all of the tools provided if you give yourself permission to see things from a new perspective at least for the duration of this book. Fully embrace the practice of not only learning about and understanding these concepts and tools but actually working towards putting them into practice in your life as well. As you begin to see just how powerful they are and how they support you in moving forward towards a more positive future, you will quickly begin to realize why they matter so much.

Lastly, there is one major concept that you need to realize before you begin listening this book. That is — self-compassion is an act of self-care, but it is also a tool that is learned through personal development practices. You are not going to be able to achieve self-compassion all in one attempt, nor will you truly be able to measure or grade yourself on the level of self-compassion that you currently have or that you develop. While there are ways for you to track your improvements and we will go into detail on those ways later, you need to understand that this practice is solely about helping yourself feel better and feel more positive in your approach to life. By allowing yourself to embody that balance, you will begin to feel far more peaceful overall.

Now, if you are ready to embark on the next chapter of your journey in self-development, it is time that you begin! Remember, self-compassion is a powerful tool for you to equip yourself with, so approach this book as open-mindedly as you possibly can. And of course, enjoy the process!

Chapter 1: Understanding the Self

Your Self or your identity is an important element of who you are. When you consider who you are, the illusion that you come up with is how you identify yourself. Although we tend to believe that our selves are an inherent part of who we are and that our personal beliefs over ourselves are finite and final, the reality is that who we are and who we think we are, typically reflect two entirely different people. Many people fail to realize that there is a difference and often find themselves genuinely believing that they are the person whom they envision in their minds and that there is no other alternative or option. As a result, they may end up developing a highly toxic, unrealistic, and self-sabotaging image or belief around who they are.

Realizing that who you truly are and who you think you are is two different people can come as a sense of relief to many. When you discover that there is a good chance that you do not actually align with the images or beliefs you have created, you realize that there is an opportunity for you to see yourself in a new light. You may even get the opportunity to start seeing yourself more clearly for who you really are, rather than for the illusion that you have been holding onto in your mind. In fact, by detaching from the strict identity you have held onto in your mind, you can give yourself the opportunity to begin experiencing far more compassion towards yourself in your life.

Identity is a rather complex topic that extends far beyond the image we carry of ourselves and the image that other's carry. In fact, there is an entire psychological study devoted to understanding identity and your sense of self and helping you discover exactly "who" you are. This field of study is known as social science and is comprised of psychologists and researchers who are actively seeking to understand identity to an even deeper level and get a clear sense of what makes a person's identity. Because there are so many different levels of identity, the study itself is quite expansive and continues to discover what one's true identity is versus the way they identify themselves and the way others identify them. In the following sections, you are going to get a deeper insight into what your sense of self truly is, how it is made up, and how your sense of self impacts the way you live your life.

Discovering the Multiple Selves

There are two ways that people have multiple sense of self. The first way that you can experience multiple senses of self comes from how you interact with the people around you and the identity you possess around these people. For example, the self you are around your friends is likely quite different from the self you are around your family or your co-workers. Your environment is a huge factor in which role you will play, depending on where you are and who you are actively surrounded by. The second way that you experience multiple social selves is determined between the way you perceive yourself and the way others perceive you. Since everyone has had their own unique interactions and experiences with you, it is not unreasonable to realize that everyone sees you slightly different from how others see you. For example, your best friend may see you completely different from how your other friends may see you, or your Grandma may carry a completely different belief of who you are compared to the rest of the world. The relationship that people share with you, the experiences that you share together, and their perception of you and of people in general will all impact how people identify you. As a result, you actually have multiple identities – and no, that does not mean that you are having an identity crisis or that you have something wrong with you. It is actually entirely normal to have many identities.

When it comes to identifying yourself, you must realize that on a psychological front, you are not identifying yourself as one person inhabiting one body. You are identifying yourself based on the actual identity that you carry or the characteristics and personality traits that you are perceived to have. Your "self" is the conscious aspect of you that interacts with the world around you, communicates with other people, and shares experiences with others. Although there is no scientific evidence that proves that there is an out-of-body "self," most psychologists believe that the self is not attached to or identified by a person's body. Instead, it is the dimension of you that exists in your mind or the aspects of you that make up "who" you are beyond your physical and biological self.

This part of yourself that is not defined by your body or biology is typically described in three related but separable domains when it comes to psychological understanding. This means that there are three elements that coincide to make up your "self" or your identity. The first domain is known as your experiential self which is also known as the 'theatre of consciousness.' This part of yourself is identified as your first-person sense of being or how you personally experience the world around you. This part of yourself remains consistent over periods of time which results in psychologists believing that it is very closely linked to your memory. The second part of your identity is what is known as your private self-consciousness. This is your inner narrator or the voice that verbally narrates what is happening in your life to you privately within your mind. When you are reading, learning, or interpreting the world around you, this voice is actively narrating how you are interpreting that information and what sense you are making of it. This is the part of you that carries your beliefs and values about how the world works. Neuroscientist Antonio Damasio calls your private self-consciousness your autobiographical self because it is regularly narrating your autobiography in your mind. The third and final dimension of your identity is your public self or your persona. This is the image that you attempt to project to others through your actions, attitudes, behaviors, and words. This is the part of your self that other people interact with and see which results in this being the part of yourself that people generate perceptions around. It is through your persona that people determine what your identity is according to them and their own understanding.

With all that being said, the multiple selves that you embody comes from the persona that you share with others. People will then generate perceptions around who you are, what your identity is, and how they feel about that. It is through this persona that people will decide if they can relate to you, if they like you, and anything else relating to how they feel about you. In realizing that people generate their perceptions of you based off of one single aspect of who you truly are, it helps you realize that their perspective is not accurate. In fact, neither is yours. No one, including yourself, *truly* knows who you actually are. Everything is just generated based on beliefs, values, perspectives, and understandings that have been accumulated through varying life experiences.

Relationship with Ourselves

The relationship that you share with yourself often develops somewhere between the first and second dimensions of your identity. The way you interpret and interact with the world around you, combined with your beliefs and values helps you generate a sort of self-awareness that allows you to begin determining what you believe your identity is. Again, just like with other people, your identity is largely based off of your perception and understanding of the world around you and how it works. Even if your own perception is rarely accurate when compared to who you actually are which is a unique blend of all three layers of your dimensional identity.

Because your relationship with yourself is largely defined by your beliefs and values and your ability to live in alignment with them or not, it is easy to realize that how you identify yourself can be easily shifted based on your perceptions. If you carry certain core beliefs about how people should live, for example, and you are not living in alignment with those beliefs, then you may generate a perception that identifies you as someone who is bad or unworthy. You might relate yourself to the identities you have mentally designed for other people in society who you believe to be bad too which can result in you seeing yourself in an extremely negative light. If you carry certain core beliefs about how people should live and you *are* living in alignment with them, you may praise yourself and see yourself as good and special. You might then find yourself relating more to people in society who you see as good and positive, thus allowing you to cast yourself in a positive light.

The reality is that none of us are truly inherently good or bad, we are all just perceiving, experiencing, and responding to the world around us. Generating internal images of what is positive and what is not only results in you setting standards for yourself on how you should behave. If these standards are beyond what you can reasonably achieve or do not align with what you genuinely want in life, then you may find yourself adhering to beliefs and values that are actually rather destructive. Instead of helping you live a life of contentment and satisfaction, you may find these beliefs leading to you constantly feeling incapable and under confident. As a result, your relationship with yourself may deteriorate because the way in which you view yourself is not reasonable or compassionate.

Everyone Has Their Own Filters and Explanatory Styles

To help you develop your understanding of how your perception of yourself varies from other's perception of you, let's discuss personal filters and explanatory styles. Understanding why everyone has such different views of the world allows you to have a stronger understanding as to why there are so many aspects of your identity based on your own personas and the way that people perceive them and you. The concept of personal filters and explanatory styles is simple. A personal filter is how you see the world and your explanatory style is how you explain it to yourself and to others.

Every single person has a unique filter and explanatory style that is based on their own unique experiences in life. All of the interactions they have had, the situations they have encountered, and things they have been told by the people around them shape the way that they view life itself. How each of these small yet impactful things come together will shape how each person perceives the world around them, others that cohabit the planet with them, and themselves. So, for example, if someone along the way has learned that not washing your dishes every day is a sign of laziness and ignorance, then that person is going to believe that anyone who leaves dishes in the sink overnight is somehow "bad," including themselves.

The foundation of a person's filters and explanatory styles are rooted in childhood when a child is not yet able to generate their own independent thoughts and beliefs. Until we are six years old, our ability to critically think about things and generate our own opinions independent of the opinions of others is virtually non-existent so we absorb everything we learn. This means that anything your parents said, people around you were saying, or you were shown through other's behaviors and actions were anchored into your mind as the foundation of your personal beliefs and values. Even though you gained the capacity to think critically and start generating your own opinions around six years old, you were still actively internalizing what everyone told you because, in most cases, no one ever taught you otherwise. As a result, you likely have many different beliefs and values that stemmed in your childhood which have gone on to impact you for years to come. In fact, these very beliefs and values are believed to make up a lot of what your autobiographical-self narrates to yourself on a daily basis, thus shaping the way you see yourself. See, who you think you are may not even be an accurate reflection of how *you* think, it may actually be an internalization based on the beliefs and values you were taught by people as you were growing up.

Since every single person will hear different things throughout their lives even if they are raised in similar environments, the way that every person views and interprets the world around them varies. Even siblings will grow up to have different perceptions and beliefs based on the way that they have internalized the beliefs they heard and were shown throughout their lifetimes. It is through this process that each person develops their own personal filters and explanatory styles for how they interpret and explain the world around them. Because of this, we can conclude that any beliefs that you have around who you are and any beliefs that others have around who you are do not actually define who you truly are. Instead, they define the belief systems that you have established throughout your life until this point.

When you realize that your beliefs are what shape your *perception* of your identity and not your identity itself, it becomes a lot easier for you to have compassion for yourself. You begin to realize that how you see yourself is not necessarily a true reflection of who you are, but instead a way that you have been lead to view yourself. This view was designed to support you in feeling connected to your 'tribe' or family and community, but in some cases, it can become destructive and result in you feeling deeply disconnected from yourself. When that happens, realizing that you are not inherently 'bad' or 'wrong' because you do not feel like you fit in makes it a lot easier for you to have compassion for your feelings and for the experiences you are going through. As a result, healing from these painful emotions and moving forward into a more self-compassionate and self-loving future becomes a lot easier for you.

Thank you, this preview in now finished.

If you enjoyed this preview of my book "The Mindful Path to Self-Compassion" by Frank Steven, be sure to check out the full book on Amazon.com

Thank you.

WEIGHT LOSS AFFIRMATIONS:
Program Your Brain Daily to Lose Weight Naturally

Condition Your Body and Mind with Inspiring Affirmations to Cease Bad Habits and Stay Healthy in Just 7 Days

Table of Contents

Introduction 107
Stay Fit Affirmations 108
Weight Loss Affirmation 120
Healthy Body Affirmations 124
Healthy Eating Affirmations for Weight Loss 136
Naturally Lose Weight Affirmations 141
I AM Affirmations for Healthy Body 145
I AM Affirmations for Health #2 151
Powerful Weight Loss Affirmations 153
Affirmations for a Healthy Body 154
Confidence Affirmations 163
Condition Your Mind Affirmations 177
Affirmations for Conditioning the Body 182
Success Affirmation 191

Introduction

Congratulations on purchasing Rapid Weight Loss, Fat Burn and Calorie Blast with Powerful Affirmations and thank you for doing so!

The following chapters will provide you with Subliminal Affirmations to Condition Your Mind and Body to Naturally Lose Weight. It will help you to Look Amazing, Stay Fit and Healthy for Life.

Thanks again for choosing this audiobook! Every effort was made to ensure it is full of as much useful information as possible. Please enjoy!

Stay Fit Affirmations

- Breathing in, I feel healthy. Breathing out, I AM healthy.
- Step by step and rep by rep, I am creating my ideal body!
- Today I choose health and wellness over illness in my life.
- I am fit! I am healthy! I am strong!
- When I eat right, I feel right!
- The more water I drink the better I feel!
- My life is what I make of it and today I choose to make it healthy place to be.
- No sugar for me! My immune system is healthy, strong, and protecting me right now!
- When I feel good, I exercise. When I exercise, I feel good.
- Today and every day, I cleanse my being with the life force of my breath.
- I AM healthy in mind, body, and spirit!
- My body is a marvelous machine that supports and meets my every need!
- Day by day, my body is transforming into the vision I have for it.
- Today I am healthy, strong, and disease-free!
- I am strong, vibrant, and healthy!
- Today and every day, I express my gratitude for my good health.
- Today I am blessed by the beautiful and delicious food that brings me to full health!
- My pain is limited to my body. I am constantly connected to something far greater than my body.

- As my reasons for holding on to my excess weight melt away, so does the weight.
- Today I am shedding the pounds as I shred my self doubt.
- Today nothing, and I mean nothing, stands between me and my goal weight. I am there before I know it!
- Day by day, I am losing the weight and the people around me are taking notice.
- My heart beats strong and healthy!
- My lungs breathe clear and strong!
- Day in and day out, I develop the habits of health!
- My body is the very picture of health and vitality!
- Today I am shedding pounds as i shred my self-doubt!
- My body is a well-oiled machine ready to meet my every need!
- I pay attention to the needs of my body. I feed it, exercise it, and love it!
- Today I push my limits in the gym so that tomorrow I can push the limits in my life!
- Today my own well-being is my top priority.
- Today I love my body fully, deeply and joyfully.
- My body has its own wisdom and I trust that wisdom completely.
- My body is simply a projection of my beliefs about myself.
- I am growing more beautiful and luminous day by day.
- I choose to see the divine perfection in every cell of my body.
- As I love myself, I allow others to love me too.
- Flaws are transformed by love and acceptance.
- Today I choose to honor my beauty, my strength and my uniqueness.
- I love the way I feel when I take good care of myself.

- Today I am transforming my body into calorie-burning machine.
- As my self-confidence rises, the number on the scale drops!
- Who I am transcends a number on a scale! Today I focus on my health not my weight!
- Today I experience vibrant health and profound well-being!
- Even at the height of my pain, I experience moments of release, contentment, and joy.
- I may have to live with pain, but I absolutely refuse to be defined by it!
- I love and accept myself at my current weight, even as I march pound by pound to my goal weight!
- My contributions to life measure my self-worth not the scale!
- Happiness is an attitude not a number on a scale! I refuse to be defined by my weight!
- I beyond the need for food to fill me up. My life is full of people and activities that do it.
- I cannot lose 100 pounds this week, but I CAN lose three pounds and I AM!
- Today I see myself at my goal weight. I feel my feelings at my goal weight. I see the clothes I wear. I see the experiences I have. I hear the compliments I receive. Today I am my goal weight. Today I am my goal weight. Today I am my goal weight.
- Day by day, I am transforming my body into a high performance machine!
- My weight loss is within me. My diet is only a tool to get me to my goal.
- As I commit to my exercise program, I transform my body!

- Step by step and rep by rep, I am losing pounds and inches today!
- A fit, healthy person lives within me. Today that person emerges.
- Today I eat for my goal weight! Today I exercise for my goal weight! Today I AM my goal weight!
- The more I bike the better I feel and the better I feel the more I bike!
- The more I run, the better I feel and the better I feel the more I run!
- I am slender, strong, and perfectly conditioned.
- The longer I exercise the stronger I get and the stronger I get the longer I exercise!
- I am an immaculate being of light. Perfect in form and function. My body is a marvelous machine that supports and meets my every need.
- My weight is meaningless in the big picture. Today I release the need to weigh one pound more than I want to!
- Pound by pound, inch by inch, choice by choice I am becoming healthy and fit!
- I struggle, but I grow. I fall, but I get up. Even amid adversity, I keep moving towards my goal weight.
- Today my portion size is shrinking and so is my waistline.
- I am beautiful, I am fit, I am healthy; and more so every day!
- Today I am making the choices and the changes to have the body I want!
- Today and every day, I feel the momentum building in my life for a healthy, fit lifestyle.
- I love my body and today I treat it with the respect it deserves.

- I deserve a healthy, fit body and today I claim it!
- Today I weigh less than yesterday and tomorrow I weigh even less!
- Today I am seeing the new, slimmer me in the mirror and I love that!
- Today I am making peace with food. Food nourishes my body, but I nourish my soul!
- All excess fat is melting away from my body.
- All my work-outs are concentrated and intense.
- As my body becomes slimmer I feel a great sense of lightness and freedom.
- Being fit and vital is one of the top priorities in my life.
- Daily exercise makes me feel fantastic!
- Daily exercise makes me healthy and attractive.
- Dancing improves my vitality and frees my soul.
- Every action I take moves me towards my perfect body.
- Every day I become more agile and lithe.
- Every day I get maximum results by increasing the intensity of my work outs.
- Every day I look slimmer and firmer.
- Every day I maximize my physical potential.
- Every day my body becomes slimmer and firmer.
- Every day my body becomes stronger and leaner.
- Every day my body becomes younger and fitter.
- Every day my muscles become stronger and more defined.
- Every day my muscles grow stronger and firmer.
- Every moment of every day I am becoming leaner and fitter.
- Every physical activity I take part in, helps me to reach my ideal weight.

- Every time I exercise I build more muscle and burn more fat.
- Exercise does as much for my mental state as it does for my body.
- Exercise greatly improves my positive self image.
- Exercise is the best stress reliever ever invented.
- Exercise makes my body feel powerful and vital.
- Exercise releases endorphins, which makes me a happier person.
- Exercise revitalizes my body and refreshes my mind.
- Exercise tones up my body and tunes up my self-esteem.
- Exercising daily gives me incredible energy.
- Exercising daily improves my mood.
- Exercising is fun and revitalizing.
- Exercising is one of my favorite stress relievers.
- Exercising is rejuvenating; it brings me abundant energy.
- I always find the time to exercise.
- I always look for opportunities to exercise my body.
- I always make the time to improve my body.
- I always stretch out my muscles after exercising.
- I am a lean, mean, muscle machine.
- I am adding healthful years to my life by exercising daily.
- I am always looking for fun new ways to stay fit.
- I am delighted with the shape and tone of my body.
- I am exceptionally agile and lithe.
- I am extremely flexible.
- I am extremely proud of my incredible figure.
- I am feeling healthier and fitter every day.
- I am feeling thinner every day.
- I am fit and trim.

- I enjoy being fit and firm.
- I am in great physical shape.
- I am in top physical condition.
- I am increasing my energy every day through regular exercise.
- I am incredibly fit and lithe.
- I am lean and toned, with well-defined muscles.
- I am often complimented on my fantastic figure.
- I am power personified.
- I am proud of how I look.
- I am proud of my outstanding physique.
- I am slender, strong, and perfectly proportioned.
- I am slim, trim and well toned.
- I am totally committed to exercise, and the results it brings.
- I am totally motivated to keep my body fit and strong.
- I am totally motivated to work out every day.
- I am very proud of my physique.
- I am willing to do whatever it takes to be fit and strong.
- I can easily see myself at my healthy weight and work daily to achieve this goal.
- I choose walking over driving whenever possible.
- I commit myself to developing the highest level of fitness in my life.
- I cycle for 20 minutes every day.
- I devote 20 minutes a day to aerobic exercise.
- I do at least one aerobic activity every day.
- I do yoga exercises every day.
- I drive less and ride more.
- I drive less and walk more.
- I easily attain my ideal weight by exercising every day.
- I enjoy going to the gym and do it regularly.

- I enjoy keeping myself fit and strong.
- I enjoy staying fit and trim.
- I enjoy working out regularly and love the energy it gives me.
- I exercise daily so my body stays fit and strong.
- I exercise regularly and it shows.
- I faithfully exercise 5 days a week.
- I feel fantastically vibrant and refreshed after exercise.
- I feel good about the way I look.
- I feel great when I exercise.
- I feel incredibly powerful and alive when I exercise.
- I feel so incredibly alive when I work out.
- I give my fitness workouts 100% effort.
- I go for long walks every day.
- I go jogging 4 times a week.
- I go running every day.
- I go to the gym three times a week.
- I have a fantastic new wardrobe to flatter my new, leaner body.
- I have a fit and attractive body.
- I have a lean, well-toned body.
- I have a powerful, lean body.
- I have a sexy body that I love creating and maintaining.
- I have all the energy and motivation I need to exercise every day.
- I have an exercise schedule that I stick to like glue.
- I have dropped two dress sizes and it feels fabulous.
- I have great stamina and resilience.
- I have the body of an athlete.
- I have the perfect figure – both shapely and strong.
- I keep myself in tiptop shape.
- I leave the car at home and walk to work today.

- I like keeping myself in great physical shape.
- I look and feel fantastic in my new fit body.
- I look and feel like a twenty-year-old athlete.
- I look good and feel great, and exercise regularly to maintain this feeling.
- I love being fit and strong.
- I love being healthy and fit.
- I love creating my dream body.
- I love exercise and use this time to feed my mind with positive thoughts and affirmations.
- I love exercise because it provides me with incredible energy.
- I love exercising and always look for new, enjoyable ways to keep in shape.
- I love how I feel after exercise.
- I love my rowing machine!
- I love pumping iron!
- I love the natural high I get from exercise.
- I love the way I feel in my new body.
- I love the way my body moves.
- I love to exercise and my body responds by performing beautifully.
- I love to feel the burn after exercise.
- I love using my exercise bike every day.
- I love using my rowing machine every day.
- I love using my treadmill every day.
- I love walking and do it often.
- I love wearing clothes that flatter my incredible figure.
- I love what regular exercise does for my body and mind.
- I love working out at my local gym.
- I never miss a workout.
- I put total effort into all my work outs.

- I raise the 'feel good' endorphin levels of my body through regular exercise.
- I really enjoy the energy that exercise gives me.
- I really love how exercising makes me feel.
- I rebound for ten minutes every day.
- I ride my bicycle to work every day.
- I speed up my metabolism by exercising regularly.
- I take brisk walks every day.
- I take full responsibility for my weight and physique.
- I take my bicycle out for a ride every day.
- I take time to exercise every day.
- I turn fat into lean muscle quickly and easily.
- I use my exercise time to listen to my affirmations.
- I use my exercise time to visualize my goals.
- I walk more and drive less.
- I work out at the gym regularly.
- It feels absolutely terrific to be able to get into my old jeans.
- It feels fantastic to have a firm, toned body.
- It is easy for me to stick to my health and fitness plan.
- It is my greatest desire to live each and every day with increased vitality.
- It is obvious that I enjoying working out daily.
- My body feels terrific!
- My body is a perfect 10.
- My body is in fantastic shape.
- My body is incredibly flexible.
- My body is strong and lithe.
- My body is trained to burn fat and build muscle.
- My body is virtually fat-free.
- My body looks and feels fantastic.
- My body looks and feels younger than my years.

- My body-fat ratio is an amazing 15 percent .
- My commitment to exercise yields fantastic results.
- My constant thoughts of physical perfection are creating the body that I desire.
- My daily fitness routine returns exceptional results.
- My daily workouts make me feel super.
- My desire to improve my fitness increases daily.
- My exercise routine yields excellent results.
- My fitness is improving by leaps and bounds.
- My fitness routine gives me outstanding results.
- My fitness routine is enjoyable and energizing.
- My fitness routine is fun and invigorating.
- My mind and body work together to create my perfect physique.
- My muscles are well defined.
- My muscles definition increases daily.
- My new leaner body gives me an incredible sense of self-esteem.
- My physical coordination improves rapidly every day.
- My running shoes and I are best friends.
- My stamina and strength increases with each step I take.
- My stomach is flat and firm and my waistline is trim.
- Physical fitness is an important part of my daily routine.
- Regular exercise guarantees me a great night's sleep.
- Regular exercise has improved my posture immensely.
- Regular exercise immensely improves my confidence and self-esteem.
- Regular exercise makes me feel great.
- Step by step and rep by rep, I am creating my perfect body.
- Taking long walks keeps me fit and gives me time to clear my mind.

- The better I feel physically, the more positive my attitude is.
- The fitter I become, the more energy I have.
- The leaner I become, the healthier I feel.
- When I exercise, my mind is free to concentrate on visualizing my goals.
- Whenever I exercise I feel rejuvenated and alive.
- While exercising, I feel healthier and healthier by the minute.
- With every breath I take, I am bringing greater and greater vitality into my life.
- With every exercise I do, my muscles get stronger and firmer.
- With every repetition, my muscles become more well-defined.

Weight Loss Affirmation

- I love and approve myself.
- I am at peace with my body, heart, and soul.
- Every day, I am feeling healthier and stronger.
- I am learning how to love my body.
- It's safe for me to be myself.
- Today, I focus on the good things that are unfolding in my life.
- Trusting my body is becoming easier and easier.
- Healing is happening in my body and in my mind.
- I choose to breathe in relaxation and breathe out stress.
- My health is improving and so is my life.
- I am surrounded and protected by the healing white light.
- Everything I eat heals me and nourishes me.
- Making small changes are becoming easier for me.
- Healing happens with each baby step I take.
- I am choosing progress over perfection.
- I am guided by my intuition. I know what to eat and how to live my life.
- I naturally connect with other like-minded, positive people.
- Letting go of the past is good for me. It is safe for me to let go.

- I can feel that everything is beginning to change.
- I am feeling healthy, focused and determined.
- Lots of new and exciting things are opening up in my life.
- I can heal my body. I am healing my body. My body is healing.
- I can do this. I am doing this. Healing is happening right now.
- I am guided by a higher power.
- I am energetic and strong.
- I see the best in everyone and they in me.
- I believe in my ability to truly love myself for who I am.
- I accept my body shape and acknowledge the beauty it holds.
- I am the creator of my future and the driver of my mind.
- I let go of unhelpful patterns of behavior around food.
- I allow myself to make choices and decisions for my higher good.
- I let go of any guilt I hold around food choices.
- I accept my body for the shape I have been blessed with.
- I let go of relationships that are no longer for my higher good.
- I believe in myself and acknowledge my greatness.
- I allow myself to feel good being me.
- I accept myself for who I am.

- I bring the qualities of love into my heart.
- I have hope and certainty about the future.
- I am grateful for the body I own and all it does for me.
- I do a healthy amount of exercise regularly.
- My body gets all the nutrients it needs.
- My desire for fattening foods is dissolving.
- I have a strong urge to eat only health-giving and nutritious foods.
- I feel good about myself.
- I am attaining and maintaining my ideal weight.
- I am strong and healthy.
- I am peaceful and calm.
- My Mind, Body & Soul are gifts of the Universe to me.
- My body is my temple that I love and takes care of every single day of my life.
- I am thin now
- I have a great body
- I am slim and beautiful
- I visualize my ideal body and take action to make it happen
- I am dedicated to achieving my ideal weight
- I believe deeply in my ability to be thin and healthy
- I am dedicated to losing weight
- My mind is focused on achieving my weight loss goals
- I always watch what I eat
- I am naturally thin
- Each day I become thinner and more fit

- I will reach my weight loss goals
- I will have the body I've always wanted
- I am becoming more focused on losing weight
- I am finding it easier to envision weight loss success
- Others are beginning to notice how thin and healthy I am
- Eating right and losing weight is becoming easier and easier
- I am coming closer to achieving my ideal body
- I am transforming into someone who is thin, healthy, and happy
- I will become thin and set a good example for others
- I am naturally thin
- I love my body
- I have total belief in myself
- I visualize my ideal body and this motivates me to keep losing weight
- I deserve to be thin
- I have the power to achieve a high degree of health and well-being
- I will nurture and respect my body always
- My mind is totally attuned to my body
- Being thin and healthy is very important
- It feels great to lose weight and get in shape

Healthy Body Affirmations

- I am motivated to exercise
- I always stick to my exercise plan
- I always finish all my exercises
- I am naturally driven to get in shape and be the healthiest I can be
- I exercise every day and I love it
- I am always motivated to exercise
- I stay motivated through out my entire workout routine

- I am in great shape because I never miss a workout
- I always look forward to exercising
- I am totally focused on getting myself in shape
- I will motivate myself to exercise
- I am becoming more and more motivated to exercise
- I am changing into someone who is always motivated to exercise
- I will exercise even when I don't feel like it
- I will exercise every day and achieve the body of my dreams
- I am finding it easier to motivate myself to exercise
- I will always finish my workout no matter how tired I am
- Others are beginning to notice how dedicated I am to getting in shape
- I am transforming into someone who exercises regularly and is in great shape
- I am starting to go to the gym every day
- I am naturally motivated to exercise
- The motivation to exercise comes naturally to me
- I love exercising

- I am totally focused on sticking to my workout routine and getting in shape
- My motivation to exercise is helping me to achieve optimum health
- I find it easy to get pumped up about going to the gym every day
- I am naturally driven to get in shape
- I am the kind of person who just loves pushing myself during my workout
- It feels great when I exercise regularly and take care of myself
- Keeping myself in top shape is extremely important to me
- I only eat healthy food
- I eat at regular intervals throughout the day
- I easily choose healthy snacks over junk
- I eat lots of fruits and vegetables
- I always eat a balanced meal
- I am a disciplined eater
- I always make sure to eat breakfast
- I eat healthy to energize my mind and my body
- I am dedicated to eating healthy foods every day
- I am focused on providing proper nutrition to my body
- I will only eat healthy food
- I am becoming a healthy eater
- Others are beginning to notice that I always eat healthy
- I am getting healthier thanks to my healthy eating habits
- I will continue to improve the quality of my diet
- I will always eat vegetables at every meal
- Eating healthy is becoming easier
- I am starting to eat more moderately sized meals
- I am starting to enjoy the taste of fruits and vegetables

- I will always choose nutritious food over junk
- I enjoy fruits and vegetables
- I fuel my body with only the best foods
- I find it easy to eat a healthy diet
- I am a natural healthy eater
- I love vegetables
- Others see me as someone who is health conscious and in control of their diet
- I am relaxed.
- I am peaceful & calm.
- I feel good.
- My body naturally sheds unneeded fat.
- I have full ability to control my weight.
- My appetite is easily satisfied with a small amount of food.
- My body gets all the nutrients it needs.
- My body is dissolving excess fat for it no longer needs it.
- I am strong and healthy.
- My appetite for fattening foods has dissolved.
- I see myself slender, fit, and trim.
- I am easily satisfied with meals.
- I am calm and relaxed when I eat.
- I have tremendous self-control to hold to my diet.
- I have a strong urge to eat only health-giving and nutritious foods.
- I feel good about myself.
- My body is strong and healthy.
- I take good care of my body.
- I do a healthy amount of exercise regularly.
- I like myself.
- I have perfect control of my weight.
- I refuse junk food.

- I eat healthy foods only.
- I love nutritious foods.
- I am attaining and maintaining my ideal weight.
- I make sure to eat meals at the same time every day
- I enjoy eating healthy food
- I always start my day off by eating something healthy
- Nutrition is very important to my quality of life
- I am beautiful
- I love my body
- I have a healthy body image
- I accept myself completely
- I am thankful for my body
- I am building a positive body image
- My body is perfect just the way it is
- I am confident in the way I look
- I always feel comfortable in my own skin
- I appreciate my body
- I will have a healthy body image
- I will always love my body no matter what
- I am beginning to accept myself more and more
- I am beginning to feel content with the way I look
- I am becoming happier with my body
- Each day I look and feel better
- I will always have gratitude for my body
- My self acceptance is beginning to change the way other people see me
- I am overcoming negativity and building a positive attitude towards myself
- I am finding it easier to feel confident in the way I look
- Having a healthy body image comes naturally to me
- Feeling positive about my body is normal for me
- I naturally love and accept my body

- Whenever I look in the mirror I always see something positive
- Having a healthy body image improves the quality of my life
- I deserve to be confident and happy
- Self acceptance comes naturally to me
- I find it easy to think positively about my body
- People are drawn to me because I am confident in the way I look
- My body is beautiful and I respect it deeply
- I am in control of my hunger
- I have power over my stomach
- I know when to stop eating
- I resist eating temptations
- I avoid overeating
- I eat proper proportions
- I eat only when I have to
- I am a healthy eater
- I am only hungry at meal times
- I watch what I eat
- I will stop feeling hungry
- I will focus on my food intake
- I am becoming a healthy eater
- Others see me as lean and in shape
- I will develop an intuition for when I am full
- I will only eat when I need to
- Hunger will not bother me
- I will restrain myself from eating too much
- I will stop feeling the need to eat
- I will live a healthier lifestyle
- I naturally know when to stop eating
- I always put down my fork when I'm full

- My body tells me when I'm full
- My hunger diminishes when I want it to
- I am naturally intuitive about my food intake
- I have always been in control of my hunger
- My hunger naturally subsides after I've eaten enough
- I enjoy eating healthy food
- I always take care of my body
- I am able to control what I eat and when I eat it
- I am comfortable with my body
- I like how I look
- I am good enough for myself
- I enjoy being healthy
- I am in shape
- I exercise for myself, not for anyone else
- I have healthy eating habits
- I exercise regularly
- I am lean and fit
- I work hard at staying healthy
- I will stay healthy
- I will take care of my body
- I will stop feeling physically insufficient
- I will be satisfied with my body
- I will work hard to stay in shape
- I will pursue my positive vision of my body
- I am becoming a healthier eater
- I will be content with my body shape
- I will exercise regularly
- I will stop feeling self-conscious about my body
- I have always been healthy
- I love eating healthy foods
- I am intuitive to what my body needs
- I was born with a high metabolism

- I always make healthy choices
- I am naturally persistent with my healthy eating
- I love exercising
- I love my body
- I am always comfortable with my appearance
- I have a perfect body shape for me
- I am healthy
- My mind is positive and healthy
- My body is strong and healthy
- I always eat healthy food
- I exercise and take care of my body
- I am dedicated to improving my health
- I am resilient against illness
- I recover quickly from being sick
- My immune system is strong
- I always make healthy choices
- I will improve my health
- I will strengthen my body
- I will think positively about my health
- Each day I become stronger
- I am beginning to feel healthier and more energetic
- I am transforming into someone who has perfect health
- I am starting to enjoy eating healthy foods
- Every day I find it easier to make healthy choices
- I will achieve abundant health
- I will become totally focused on healthy living
- I am naturally healthy
- I can beat any health challenge
- I have a healthy mind body connection
- Overcoming illness is easy for me
- Feeling healthy and strong is normal
- I have vibrant health

- Others see me as someone who lives a healthy lifestyle
- It is important that I eat right and exercise
- I enjoy eating healthy food
- I have a positive attitude towards my health
- I exchange high fat foods for high energy foods and all excess fat is now being removed from me.
- For me, eating and emotional comfort are separate and I forgive myself for overeating.
- I let go of all reasons and excuses for not eating healthy meals.
- I replace dieting with healthy eating principles and habits.
- Healthy eating and I are one and I am richly rewarded for my healthy eating habits.
- I accept healthy eating as a way of life.
- I only eat the foods that are good for me.
- I eat the right foods at the right times.
- I refuse to let other people influence me to eat too much.
- I can eat right without hurting anyone's feelings.
- I am allowed to decline food and do so in total peace.
- The Universe provides more than enough food for me.
- I willingly keep my meal portions small.
- I choose fruits and vegetables over salty, sugary high fat foods every time.
- Fresh vegetables feel and taste good in my mouth.
- I get all the vitamins and nutrients I need.
- I believe in my ability to love and accept myself for who I am.
- I set myself free from all the guilt I carry around the food I chose in the past.
- Every day I am exercising and taking care of my body.
- Healing is happening in both my body and mind.

- Every time I inhale, fresh energy fills my entire being and every time I exhale, all toxins and body fat leave my body.
- My health is improving more and more every day, and so is my body.
- Everything I eat heals and nourishes my body, which helps me reach the ideal weight.
- I am closer and closer to my ideal weight with each and every day.
- I can do this, I am doing this, my body is losing weight right now.
- I am letting go of any guilt I hold around food.
- Eating healthy foods helps my body get all of the nutrients it needs to be in best shape.
- I am closer and closer to my ideal weight with each and every day.
- I feel my desire for fat-rich foods dissolving.
- I have a strong urge to eat only healthy foods, and let go of any processed foods.
- I am the best version of myself, and I am working hard to become even better. I will lose weight because I want to, and I have the power to do this.
- My body is my temple, and I attentively take care of it every day by eating only healthy foods that heal and nourish me.
- I am aware that my metabolism is working in my advantage by helping me in gaining my optimal weight.
- I am attaining and maintaining my desired weight.
- I have the power to easily control my weight through a combination of healthy eating and exercising.
- I am grateful to my body for all the things it does for me.
- Every cell in my body is healthy and fit, and so am I.

- I feel my body losing weight in every single moment of the day.
- I always chew my food properly so that my body can digest it and take out the nutrients I need to lose weight.
- I believe in my ability to change my habits and create new, positive ones.
- I no longer feel the urge to stuff my body with unhealthy foods, and I can easily resist temptations.
- I enjoy life by staying fit and maintaining my ideal weight.
- I am capable of achieving my weight loss goals, and I will not let anything stay in my way until then.
- I accept my body exactly the way it is and I constantly work on improving it.
- I completely understand that unhealthy foods do not help me lose weight, so I eat only healthy, nutritious foods.
- My metabolism rate is at its optimum level, and this helps me reach my ideal body weight.
- I love fruits and vegetables and eat them every day
- I am determined to make exercise and healthy eating my daily lifestyle.
- I crave clean, nutritious and healthy food that keeps me fueled and energized, not lethargic and dull.
- I make healthy eating choices daily in order to treat my mind, body, and spirit well.
- Eating Well Expresses Itself In My Chronically Excellent Health
- I eat clean several times a day and drink lots of water, i lose weight with ease
- I eat healthy, nutritious and digestible food every day.
- I AM FIT I AM STRONG I AM HEALTHY.
- I will eat healthy balance meal.

- I will learn to love and appreciate my new dietary restrictions
- I am happy with the idea that I can easily and comfortably wean myself off the behaviors of eating too much in the evenings as a boredom-coping mechanism. I can learn far better patterns!
- It is really becoming quite easy for me, to eat calorie dilute foods frequently and pleasurably. I eat beets and broccoli, and I enjoy eating raw carrots, and raw bell peppers.
- It is fun for me to think about having a week or so under my belt, as far as doing well at hunger-based eating, and being well-established in my new habits. This feels good to have such success!
- My food choices are very intelligent choices. I know when it is a good time to give my body some food, and I know how to do other things, when food is not the answer.
- My food intake is a personal choice, and I really don't follow any particular health guru on every matter. I take nutritional guidelines under advisement, and decide what is best for me right now.
- My health is my strength. I have a lean body, and I have a lot of wonderful energy. My energy is positive, and I enjoy eating a lot of leafy greens each week.
- This is the first time in my life that I have eaten a steady diet of leafy greens, and I really do find that it's nourishing and satiating.
- I don't really need to convince anyone else that what I'm doing and how I'm eating, is good for my figure. The outcomes are obvious. Maybe there are other ways to be lean and sexy, but I have found one reliable way, and I feel good about that.

- My heart is happy and I am positioning myself to be confident at anything I pursue -- confident as a runner, confident as a dancer, confident as a sexual partner, confident in any outfit. You name it!

Healthy Eating Affirmations for Weight Loss

- Controlling my appetite is easy for me now.
- Eating healthy foods makes me look and feel better.
- Every day I become a more nutrition-conscious cook.
- Every day I get closer to my idea weight.
- Everything I do moves me to closer health.
- Everything I eat helps to make my body strong and healthy.
- Feelings of confidence and comfort come from my thoughts, not from food.
- Healthy foods help my brain think with greater clarity.
- I always choose the most nutritional foods.
- I always eat healthy foods when I'm at work.
- I always ensure that I get my 5-a-day every day!
- I always savor the flavor when eating.
- I am always open to trying new health-giving foods.
- I am effortlessly maintaining my perfect body weight.
- I am forever grateful for the abundance of nourishing foods I have to choose from.
- I am getting closer to my perfect weight every day.
- I am in total control of my cravings and only indulge those that are healthy.
- I am maintaining my ideal body weight easily and effortlessly now.
- I am my ideal weight of…
- I am only interested in eating nutrition-rich foods.
- I am open to trying new foods.
- I am so excited that I now weigh…
- I am thankful for the bounty of health-giving food that nature provides.
- I am what I eat; I therefore only eat the very best.

- I buy more raw foods and leave the packaged foodstuffs at the store.
- I buy only the most nutritious, health-giving foods.
- I choose to eat healthy meals every day.
- I choose to eat smaller portions at every meal.
- I control my weight through healthy eating and regular exercise.
- I digest my food with ease and efficiency.
- I do everything I need to do to achieve my healthy weight.
- I do everything necessary to maintain a healthy weight.
- I drink eight glasses of fresh spring water every day.
- I drink plenty of water to stay healthy and hydrated.
- I easily let go of all unhealthy eating habits.
- I easily let go of unhealthy food cravings.
- I easily maintain my ideal weight of….
- I easily maintain my perfect weight.
- I easily resist all temptation to eat empty foods.
- I eat a healthy and balanced diet.
- I eat a well balanced diet of health-sustaining foods.
- I eat all the right foods for optimum health and energy.
- I eat exactly the right amount of food for my body's needs.
- I eat health giving fruits and vegetables every day.
- I eat healthy and nutritious foods at every meal.
- I eat healthy foods and enjoy regular exercise.
- I eat healthy foods that are good for my body.
- I eat light and feel light.
- I eat moderate proportions of healthy, nutritious foods.
- I eat my food slowly, chewing each bite thoroughly and savouring it's wonderful flavour.
- I eat only when necessary.

- I eat six small, healthy meals every day.
- I eat slowly and mindfully.
- I eat slowly and savor every bite.
- I eat the right foods in the right amounts.
- I eat to live, not live to eat.
- I eat what is best for my health and well-being.
- I effortlessly maintain my ideal weight.
- I effortlessly remove fat from my body by eating only fat-free foods.
- I enjoy eating balanced, nutritious meals.
- I enjoy eating foods that my body needs to be healthy.
- I enjoy eating smaller portions and taking the time to appreciate the taste.
- I enjoy the taste of fresh fruits and vegetables.
- I ensure that I only eat the most health-giving foods.
- I ensure that my body receives all the vitamins and nutrients it needs.
- I ensure that my calorie intake does not surpass my calorie expenditure.
- I feed my body healthy nutritious food.
- I feel a great sense of self-respect when I feed myself healthy, nutritious foods.
- I find it very easy to maintain my ideal weight.
- I get closer to my perfect weight every day.
- I help my body do its job by keeping fit and eating right.
- I honor my body and pay close attention to its needs.
- I keep my meal portions small and nutritious.
- I listen to my body and heed its needs.
- I look and feel lighter today.
- I love eating food that is good for me.
- I love eating foods that are good for my body.
- I love eating foods that make me healthier.

- I love eating health-giving fruits and vegetables.
- I love eating healthy raw foods.
- I love eating nutritious, health-empowering food.
- I love eating salads.
- I love my body and treat it with total respect.
- I love myself and therefore choose to watch what I eat.
- I love preparing nutritious, health-empowering meals for my family.
- I monitor my eating habits and ensure that I only consume health-giving foods.
- I now eat lots of fresh, healthy fruits and vegetables.
- I only choose to put healthy things into my body.
- I only consume healthy, nutritious foods.
- I only crave those things that are health-giving.
- I only eat foods that afford my body optimum health.
- I only eat foods that are barcode-free!
- I only eat foods that energize my body and mind.
- I only eat healthy foods in healthy amounts.
- I only eat healthy, empowering foods.
- I only eat the foods that sustain my well-being.
- I only eat when I am hungry.
- I only feed my body with the healthiest foods.
- I only fuel my body with nutritious, health-promoting foods.
- I only put healthy things into my body.
- I prefer to eat meals that support my health and well-being.
- I really enjoy eating less and eating better.
- I remember to put smaller portions of food on my plate.
- I resist all temptations to eat calorie-rich desserts.
- I resist all temptations to eat fatty foods.
- I resist all temptations to eat unhealthy, junk foods.

- I shrink my appetite to a healthy size by eating a little less every day.
- I stay healthy by eating healthy.
- I stop eating before feeling full.
- I strive to avoid foods that upset my well-being.
- I take good care of my body by eating correctly.
- I train my subconscious mind to crave only those foods which nourish my body.
- I use food to build and maintain my body, not to satisfy unwanted habits.
- My body is my temple, and I treat it accordingly.
- My body is perfect because I only eat perfect foods.
- My body metabolizes food very quickly.
- My body thanks me for eating healthy, nutritious foods.
- My calorie intake is on target for my age, sex and build.
- My metabolism continuously keeps me fit and trim.
- Nothing unhealthy goes into my body.
- The healthier I eat, the better I feel.
- Water is my favorite beverage!
- When I'm comfortably full, I stop eating.

Naturally Lose Weight Affirmations

1. I love my body and I love myself.

2. I am perfect and complete just the way I am.

3. I feed my body healthy nourishing food and give it healthy nourishing exercise because it deserves to be taken care of.

4. I know the answers and solutions. I listen to myself and trust my inner judgement.

5. My brain is my sexiest body part.

6. My life is what I make of it. I have all the power.

7. My body is a vessel for my awesomeness.

8. I eat a variety of foods for my health, wellness and enjoyment.

9. There is more to life that worrying about my weight. I'm ready to experience it.

10. Food is not good or bad. It has no moral significance. I can choose to be good or bad and it has nothing to do with the amount of calories or carbohydrates I eat.

11. Being grounded and whole makes me beautiful. I can get there just by being still, breathing, listening to my intuition, and doing what I can to be kind to myself and others.

12. I deserve to be treated with love and respect.

13. Even if I don't see how amazing I am, there is someone who does. I am loved and admired.

14. I look exactly the way I'm supposed to. I know because this is the way God made me!

15. It's not about working on myself; it's about being okay with who I already am.

16. Body, if you can love me for who I am, I promise to love you for who you are.

17. My body can do awesome things.

18. My body is a gift. I treat it with love and respect.

19. Life is too short and too precious to waste time obsessing about my body. I am going to take care of it to the best of my ability and get out of my head and into the world.

20. A goal weight is an arbitrary number; how I feel is what's important.

21. As long as I am good, kind, and hold myself with integrity, it doesn't matter what other people think of me.

22. I trust the wisdom of my body.

23. I use my energy to pay attention to myself, my inner wisdom, my virtues, my path, and my journey.

24. When I look to others to dictate who I should be or how I should look, I reject who I am.

25. Accepting myself as I am right now is the first step in growing and evolving.

26. All magazine photos are airbrushed, photoshopped, and distorted.

27. I love and respect myself.

28. I enjoy feeling good. I deserve to feel good.

29. Being skinny or fat is not my identity. I am identified by who I am on the inside, a loving, wonderful person.

30. My opinion of myself is the only one that counts.

31. I am compassionate and warm. My presence is delightful to people.

32. My very existence makes the world a better place.

33. My well-being is the most important thing to me. I am responsible for taking care of me.

34. No one has the power to make me feel bad about myself without my permission.

35. I eat for energy and nourishment.

36. My needs are just as important as anyone else's.

37. Chocolate is not the enemy. It's not my friend either. It's just chocolate, it has no power over me.

38. Life doesn't start 10 pounds from now, it's already started. I make the choice to include myself in it.

39. Thighs, thank you for carrying me to where I want to go.

40. Belly, thank you for helping me digest.

41. Skin, thank you for protecting me.

42. Other people don't dictate my choices for me, I know what's best for myself.

43. I feed my body life-affirming foods so I am healthy and vital.

44. Taking care of myself feels good.

45. I choose to do and say kind things for and about myself.

I AM Affirmations for Healthy Body

- I AM nourishing my body with thoughts of abundant and radiant health

- I AM choosing All of my thoughts about my body to be healthy and positive thoughts.

- I AM sending Love to all the cells in my body, and they are now returning to their perfect original blueprint.

- I AM enjoying taking care of my precious body

- I AM enjoying a complete sense of well-being in my body and mind.

- I AM grateful for the sense of well-being that fills my consciousness every day.

- I AM allowing all aspects of my being to be vital and alive.

- I AM choosing now to love my body – it is doing it´s best to keep me healthy – My Love supports my cells to keep me healthy, vibrant and alive

- I AM now Breathing deeply to elevate my mood and energize my body.

- I AM really enjoying that All the cells in my body resonate in perfect harmony.

- I AM grateful for the aura of vibrant well-being that now surrounds my body and mind.

- I AM Divine intelligence.

- I AM Love

- I AM Harmony

- I AM Complete

- I AM proud and excited by being a person that has taken full responsibility for my health and wellbeing

- I AM enjoying that every cell in my body vibrates in the frequency of brilliant health and vitality.

- I AM now allowing Every cell in my body to replenish, repair, and celebrate my strong and flexible body.

- I AM opening my heart to Universal Love – when I give and receive love – my body is healthy

- I AM a Soul in a human body – I chose this body – It is the best body I could have for my learning experience here on earth. I choose to honor, respect and LOVE my body.

- I AM celebrating my Vibrant health.

- I AM now sending love and gratitude to every part of my body.

- I AM now opening up and welcoming an increasingly higher dose of life force to fill up my entire being.

- I AM now Healing Deeply.

- I AM now filling my body with Divine light and love.

- I AM surprising myself every day by how easy it is for me to make healthy choices.
- I AM surprising myself with new ways of thinking that really feels empowering and uplifting.
- I AM inspired and motivated to take action NOW.
- I AM now allowing myself to be totally in sync with life. Everything that happens has a deeper meaning.
- Life is love.
- I am love
- I am willing to see life through the lens of love
- I AM bathing in energy and vitality.
- I AM nourishing my body with plenty of water
- I AM so happy and grateful for Every fiber of my being is vibrantly alive.
- I AM now surprising myself with how motivated I am to exercising
- I AM having fun while exercising my awesome body.
- I AM now working out in the way that gives me the most joy
- I AM motivated and inspired to make the choices that I know are for my highest good

- I AM enjoying my constant improvement in whatever I choose to do.

- I AM breathing more deeply because it detoxes me faster than anything else.

- I AM making the best choices for me because I CAN

- I AM walking like I mean it.

- My body posture reflects my positive mindset. I am raising my vibration just by raising my posture.

- I choose to be proud of my uniqueness.

- I am a beautiful being.

- I AM now absorbing the infinite life force from creation through the pores of my skin.

- No matter where I am, or who I am with, or which hour it is – I AM making choices that support my well being at all levels. My wellbeing and health are my top priority – so making good choices are easy and feels amazing!

- I AM curious and excited as I AM now listening to my body as it communicates clearly its wants and needs.

- Universal wisdom is flowing through my body. It is connected to something much bigger than myself.

- I AM grateful for the brilliant flexibility and awesome strength in my core muscles and joints.

- I AM grateful to have such a good friend as my body.

- I am a beautiful expression of life. I am smiling more and more without any reason, because it makes me feel good I AM now in the moment. I AM pure lifeforce in a human body.

- I AM soaring with Prana.

- I AM absorbing the life-giving energy of the universe.

- I AM Health

- I AM Wellbeing

- I AM Complete

- I AM enjoying the foods that are best for my body.

- I AM continually discovering new ways to improve my health.

- I AM returning my body to optimal health by giving it what it needs on every level.

- I AM now allowing myself to be entirely in sync with life.

- I AM allowing the intelligence of my body to do its healing work naturally now.

- I AM balancing my life between work, rest, and play.

- I AM grateful to be alive today. It is my joy and pleasure to live another wonderful day.

- I AM lovingly taking care of my body, and my body appreciates how I take care of it.

- I AM lovingly do everything I can to assist my body in maintaining perfect health.

- I AM Divinely guided to make the choices that support a robust, healthy and happy body.

- I AM now connecting to my subconscious blueprint of Perfect health.

- I AM shining the light of Perfect health and Divine intelligence.

- I AM Filling my mind with pleasant, uplifting and empowering thoughts.

- I AM now really aware that My happy thoughts help create my healthy body.

- I AM connected with that part of myself that knows how to heal.

- I AM breathing deeply and fully. I take in the breath of life, and I am nourished.

- I AM safe

- I AM free

- I AM love

- I AM continously learning new things that enhances my health and well being. Life is truly a journey.

- I AM very conscious of which foods are for my highest good. I really enjoy to be awake and alive. I am taking full responsibility of my vibration, because I am the Soul who lives in my body.

I AM Affirmations for Health #2

- I am filled with vitality, energy, and physical stamina.

- I project the white light through my body to aid me in restoring health, vitality, and youthful beauty to my entire system.

- The perfect life power that flows through every living being is now animating and vitalizing every cell and function of my physical being.

- I think, speak, and act nothing but perfect health.

- May the abundance of my Higher Self fill my mind, soul, and body with the love that brings healing in every manner.

- The divine love of my Higher Self will eradicate any desires that would hinder my body from being physically fit.

- I am perfect, I am whole, I am loved; my body is loved.

- Be merciful, Supreme Intelligence, in my hour of need for my body, my mind, my soul. Heal my every weakness through my Higher Self that makes me alive in you.

- Keep me in the way, Higher Self, that will bring healing, understanding, and a righteous heart in all my days.

- I do not accept this condition The Infinite Intelligence's plan for me is perfect health, free of pain. I am healed and I accept this healing now.

- My body is the temple of the living Lord. I am filled with the Infinite Intelligence of God who sees this body only as whole and perfect. I do not accept this diagnosis of incurable disease. I am a perfect child of God and I manifest His perfection now.

- Through the presence of my Higher Self within me, I can do all things. There is no limit to the healing power that is surging through me and healing me now.

- I claim the healing power that expresses itself in me in all ways.

- Nothing that is not of health and wholeness can get hold of me. I claim that good now in my life.

- I am perfect, I am whole, I am healthy.

- Pain or disease is of little consequence. I am Divine Intelligence.

- Divine Intelligence flows through my entire Being. Every cell in my body is revitalized with its life force.

- I am health, strength and vitality.

- I am never alone. I have the creative force within. It will help me and heal me.

- I am in partnership with the great creative intelligence.

Powerful Weight Loss Affirmations

1. I have committed myself to a healthier lifestyle.
2. I bless my food before eating it.
3. I am so grateful now that I have healthy eating habits.
4. I make wise food choices.
5. Everyday is a new beginning.
6. I am enjoying my weight release journey. This time I will complete what I started.
7. I eat in proper portions.
8. Eating healthy comes naturally to me.
9. Exercising comes naturally to me.
10. I stay focused on my ideal size.
11. I find time to exercise.
12. My metabolism rate is at its optimum and it helps me in reaching my ideal weight.
13. I love myself unconditionally.
14. Every physical movement that I make burns the extra fat in my body and helps me to maintain my ideal body weight.
15. I easily control my weight through a combination of healthy eating and exercising.
16. I love living in this beautiful body.
17. I crave food that energizes me and makes me feel good.
18. When I use my muscles I feel powerful and alive.
19. Working out releases stress and tension, the more I move the more relief I feel.
20. Food is my fuel, I give my body clean, healthy fuel.
21. I feel good inside this body.
22. This is my body, I treat it with respect and honor.
23. Healthy nutritious food is what I crave to eat.
24. I workout and see the results right away in my energy stamina and strength.
25. I am powerful, unstoppable, amazing. I can achieve my desired physique.

Affirmations for a Healthy Body

- I restore and maintain my body at optimum health.
- I am pain-free and totally in sync with life.
- I am open and receptive to all the healing energies in the Universe.
- I know that every cell in my body is intelligent and knows how to heal itself.
- I take care of my body and spirit through exercise and healthy food choices.
- I am nourished by the Universe, thus able to live a pain-free life.
- The cells in my body feel grateful to do their job obediently by keeping my body strong and healthy.
- I regularly caressing my hands, legs, and body with love to thank the cells for what they have done to my whole body. I love them.
- Until today, am a healthy and happy person.
- Healing is compassion and kindness to my body soul & spirit
- Health is at the center of all life's aspects, it is affected by all and affects all.
- I AM Healthy when my Life is in Dynamic Balance.
- I am at peace with my body, mind, heart, and soul!
- I receive healing, I am healthy and whole; all is well in my world.
- My body is a house of wellness. Each day I do something that supports wellness in my life.
- Healing happens! I get my mind out of the way and allow the intelligence of my body to do its healing work naturally.
- My wonderful body is an expression of the complete health and I love to keep it in that way.

- I lovingly do everything I can to assist my body in maintaining perfect health.
- Good health comes from love and appreciation, and I feel wonderful physically and emotionally.
- I am open and receptive to all the healing energies in the Universe.
- I know that every cell in my body is intelligent and knows how to heal itself.
- My body is always working toward perfect health.
- I now release any and all impediments to my perfect healing.
- I learn about nutrition and feed my body nourishing, wholesome food.
- I watch my thinking and only think healthy thoughts.
- I release, wipe out, and eliminate all thoughts of hatred, jealousy, anger, fear, self-pity, shame, and guilt.
- I love my body.
- I send love to each organ, bone, muscle, and part of my body.
- I flood the cells of my body with love. I accept healing and good health here and now.
- Good health comes from love and appreciation.
- As I heal my thoughts my body heals too, but more surprisingly I notice my environment becomes healthy to live in.
- My body is a perfect healing mechanism because God is in me,
- When I am filled with Love, I am naturally in a state of HEALTH & HEALING;
- The more Love I give to myself and others, the more HEALING I receive and the HEALTHIER I become.
- A healthy mind produces a healthy body.
- I deserve to be healthy, happy, and successful.

- Becoming healthier is more than losing weight. I'm going to improve the quality of my life.
- I'm going to control myself, build my discipline and not give in every time I have a craving.
- I'm going to live my life at my own pace. I don't need to try to compete with anyone else.
- I'm proud of myself for being able to turn down things that I know aren't healthy for me.
- I will invest in myself because I am worth it.
- I am good enough. I believe in myself. I am not worthless. I will heal from this.
- I'm allowed to reject toxicity.
- I'm committing myself to live a healthier life.
- My goal to lose weight is to feel healthier, happier and look better in my clothes.
- For when anxiety gets too much. "Breath in calmness, breathe out nervousness"
- I promise to work on myself every single day.
- Taking care of myself isn't selfish, it's healthy.
- My mind and body deserve to be treated better.
- One of the greatest acts of self-care is keeping the promises you make to yourself.
- Eating good foods, exercise, recovery and being around great people are simple ways to practice self-care.
- I now choose to release all anger, sorrow, frustration and emotional pain that has been building up within me.
- I open my heart to love and invite happiness, health and positive energies into my life.
- I will surround myself with a healthy environment to grow in.
- I gratefully accept all the health, wealth and happiness that the universe pours into me every day.

- love eating raw matter FROM fresh fruits like strawberries, FOR being HEALTHY with the live FORTIFYING nutrition it carries.
- I am a magnet. I attract love, health, happiness, wisdom, and wealth from the universe.
- I have everything it takes to heal completely.
- The more I embrace positivity, the healthier I am.
- My skin is clean, soft and healthy
- My body's cells know how to cure and be healthy again
- I perfectly digest food and drinks
- I'm perfectly tolerant of different weather conditions
- My body is healed quickly
- My spine is healthy and elastic
- My spine is the right
- My muscles are well built
- My vision was again perfect and lenses and glasses I do not need
- I bring as much oxygen into my body as my body is enough for the most optimal development.
- I breathe in my stomach
- I'm full of energy
- Whatever I eat or drink my body uses only the most useful materials for optimal development
- I meet new possibilities of my body
- I feel every cell of my body
- My hair is dense and quality
- My body is vital
- Consciously positively affect my health
- I'm eating healthy
- My immune system is strong
- I'm healthy
- I feel perfect in my body

- Becoming healthier is more than losing weight. I'm going to improve the quality of my life.
- I'm proud of myself for being able to turn down things that I know aren't healthy for me.
- I deserve to be healthy, happy, and successful.
- I am good enough. I believe in myself. I am not worthless. I will heal from this.
- I'm committing myself to live a healthier life.
- My goal to lose weight is to feel healthier, happier and look better in my clothes.
- My mind and body deserve to be treated better.
- Eating good foods, exercise, recovery and being around great people are simple ways to practice self-care.
- I'm not selfish if I focus on myself for a little bit. I need to make sure I'm okay and healthy.
- Self-care isn't always fun or easy but it's what I have to do to stay healthy.
- I am nurturing my body & mind with healthy foods because I love myself.
- I will surround myself with a healthy environment to grow in.
- I am a magnet for divine abundance in my health
- I enjoy the foods that are best for my body.
- I love every cell of my body.
- I make healthy choices.
- I gratefully accept all the health, wealth and happiness that the universe pours into me every day..
- I am a magnet. I attract health from the universe.
- I accept perfect health now.
- I can create fun in my life!
- I accept others just as they are and in turn,
- I am accepted just as I am.

- I want to be free.
- I am free.
- I release the fear of being the real me.
- Thank you, the universe for allowing me to walk in freedom.
- You are greatness personified, a resident genius, and a creative master.
- I am willing for all parts of my spirit to be free, and I *am* free in many areas, and becoming *more* free every day, every moment!
- I understand that change is inevitable. I welcome change and adapt myself to change.
- I think in a positive way. My thoughts create my reality.
- I envision myself wealthy in every area of my life and work toward that reality.
- I deserve to laugh. I deserve to be happy. I deserve to be loved.
- I understand that my thinking creates my experience and I now choose to use this positively in all areas of my life.
- I enjoy my duty: spreading happiness to all the people that I meet.
- I accept the things I cannot change
- I am learning something new every day
- I have entered a new, highly successful phase of my life
- I love myself first, then I love others.
- I am loving and accepting of others and this creates lasting friendships for me.
- I believe that everything's getting better and better every day.
- I am grateful for all the good things that I have in my life: joy, peace, and harmony.

- I forgive myself and understand that I'm the only one who's responsible for every situation in my life.
- I release all fears and desperation and allow love to find me.
- I always eat small portions when I am dining out.
- I always take the time to prepare healthy dinners because it makes me feel full of vitality.
- I always take the time to prepare healthy dinners when I arrive home from work because it makes me feel on top of my world.
- Even on weekends, I love sticking to structured meals and snack times, always choosing healthy foods because it makes me feel good about myself.
- I limit my indulgences to special occasions.
- If and when I am tempted to snack after dinner I always choose fruits or vegetables.
- I am always in bed by 10:00pm so that I can wake up for an early morning workout.
- I always exercise five times per week for at least 30 minutes for each session.
- Exercising always makes me feel happy, healthy and alive.
- Exercising keeps my energy, confidence and positive attitude strong.
- I am addicted to exercising, and I always find time to exercise.
- Exercise keeps me lean and trim and allows me to wear fitted clothes that make me look and feel like a million bucks!
- My muscles are strong, lean, defined and sexy.
- I work all of my muscle groups at least once per week and this keeps my figure tight and defined.

- I change my workouts every month to ensure that I'm having the most fun and that my muscles are being challenged to the max.
- I never give up on my health goals. There is no such thing as failure for me.
- Every day I am moving closer and closer to my goal.
- Every day and every week I am constantly learning new tips and tricks to enhance and protect my lean figure.
- Eating healthy and exercising nurtures my heart and soul.
- Being health conscientious gives me a competitive advantage in my career and life pursuits.
- I am worthy of good health.
- I am open to seeing everything that is no longer serving me, and I am willing to see it all with love.
- I fully accept where I am and am ready to seize this opportunity to grow.
- I focus on positive progress.
- I am supported and loved in this healing journey of mine.
- I create good health by talking and thinking about my wellness.
- I most love the parts of me that need love the most right now.
- Even though there is discomfort inside of me, I love and approve of myself.
- I am in control of the mental atmosphere I create. Thoughts can be changed and the positive thoughts I choose are helping me heal.
- I am free to be new in this moment.
- I release all negativity because it's not who I am. I make way for love because that's who I really am.

- I am a friend to my body. I forgive my body and treat it with the same loving kindness I would like to receive.
- No matter what has been or will be, my inner light can't be extinguished.
- I treat my discomfort and pain like I would an innocent child. I tend to my body with unconditional compassion and care.
- I am doing everything I can to help my body be well as quickly as possible.
- I choose thoughts that create a healthy atmosphere within and around me.
- I am a willing participant in my own wellness plan.
- I am open to new ways of improving my health.
- Every choice I make, I make it with mindfulness and a love of life. Whatever it is that I do, I love myself through it.
- I am a survivor.
- My body knows how to heal itself. I allow the intelligence of my body to move my health forward.
- I am on the path of expansion, always learning. I respect the process even when I do not understand it.
- I am so grateful to be alive. I cherish being here.
- I am willing to be with all of my thoughts and feelings without admonishing them. Instead of turning away, I stay and understand.
- I am looking for ways to express love. I am looking for beauty in the present moment. I am looking for beacons of hope everywhere I go.

Confidence Affirmations

- I am a confident person who is respected by everyone around.
- I am a unique and worthy person, and I deserve everyone's respect.
- I accept myself, and I love myself for who I am.
- It matters little what other people say. What really matters to me is how I react and what I believe in.
- My mind is filled with positive thoughts, and I understand and let go of any negative thought patterns.
- I breathe in relaxation and breathe out stress.
- I respect myself, and so do others around me.
- I choose to accept myself exactly the way I am, and be happy with my life.
- I appreciate every single thing I have in my life, and I live in absolute joy.
- I feel excitement when life brings challenges to me, and I gladly accept them without any guilt or anxiety.
- I replace "I must," "I have to" and "I should" with "I choose."
- I trust myself, and I have the confidence that I am a worthy person everyone respects.
- Meeting new people is easy. I can creative supportive relationships and make new friends without feeling anxious.
- I acknowledge both my qualities and defects, and I always strive to improve.
- I am a focused person, and I will not quit doing anything when I feel challenged or wronged.
- I am kind, loving, compassionate, and I truly care for the people around.
- I inhale self-confidence and exhale fear and anxiety.

- I have integrity, as I am a reliable person and I always do exactly what I say. Everybody can trust me.
- I trust and believe in myself, and I let go of the negative.
- Being alive makes me a happy person.
- Being myself is good and rewarding, and I always perceive challenges as opportunities to prove my abilities.
- I deserve all that is good in this world. I release any need for suffering, and I can feel happiness, confidence and love getting into my body, mind, and soul.
- I am enthusiastic and energetic, and confidence is an important part of my nature.
- I am healthy, well-groomed, and good-looking, and I acknowledge both my inner and outer beauty.
- I thrive on my absolute self-confidence. My life is beautiful, and I enjoy every single moment of it.
- I never compare myself to others, as I understand my uniqueness.
- Every time I inhale, confidence fills my entire being and every time I exhale, all guilt and shyness get washed away.
- I accept myself the way I am, and I am getting better and better in everything I do.
- I am a person who easily accepts new challenges.
- Change is inevitable and I accept it wholeheartedly.
- Losing weight comes naturally for me.
- I am happily achieving my weight loss goals.
- I am losing weight every day.
- I love to exercise regularly.
- I am eating foods that contributes to my health and wellbeing.
- I eat only when I am hungry.
- I now clearly see myself at my ideal weight.

- I love the taste of healthy food.
- I am in control of how much I eat.
- I am enjoying exercising, it makes me feel really good.
- I am becoming fitter and stronger everyday through exercise.
- I am easily reach and maintain my ideal weight
- I love and care for my body.
- I deserve to have a slim, healthy, attractive body.
- I am developing more healthy eating habits all the time.
- I am getting slimmer every day.
- I look and feel great.
- I do what it takes to be healthy.
- I am happily redefined success.
- I choose to exercise.
- I want to eat foods that make me look and feel good.
- I am responsible for my health.
- I love my body.
- I am patient with creating my better body.
- I am happily exercising every morning when I wake up so that I can reach the weight loss that I have been wanting.
- I am committing myself to my weight loss program by changing my eating habits from unhealthy to healthy.
- I am happy with every part I do in my great effort to lose weight.
- Every day I am getting slimmer and healthier.
- I am in the process of developing an attractive body.
- I am developing a lifestyle of vibrant health.
- I am creating a body that I like and enjoy.
- My lifestyle eating changes are changing my body.
- I am feeling great now that I have lost in excess of 10 pounds in 4 weeks and can't wait to meet my lady friend.
- I have a flat stomach.

- I celebrate my own power to make choices around food.
- I am happily weighing 20 pounds less.
- I am loving walking 3 to 4 times a week and do toning exercises at least 3 times a week
- I drink 8 glasses of water a day.
- I eat fruits and vegetables daily and eat mostly chicken and fish.
- I am learning and using the mental, emotional, and spiritual skills for success. I am willing to change!
- I am willing to create new thoughts about my self and my body.
- I love and appreciate my body.
- It's exciting to discover my unique food and exercise system for weight loss.
- I am weight loss success story.
- I am delighted to be the ideal weight for me.
- It's easy for me to follow a healthy food plan.
- I choose to embrace thoughts of confidence in my ability to make positive changes in my life.
- It feels good to move my body. Exercise is fun!
- I use deep breathing to help me relax and handle stress.
- I am a beautiful person.
- I deserve to be at my ideal weight.
- I am a lovable person. I deserve love. It is safe for me to lose weight.
- I am a strong presence in the world at my lower weight.
- I release the need to criticize my body.
- I accept and enjoy my sexuality. It's OK to feel sensuous.
- My metabolism is excellent.
- I maintain my body with optimal health.
- I have the perfect weight that is healthy in every ways.
- I have a height metabolic rate that is helping me burn fat everyday.
- I am always ready to visit the gym

- I have the strength for weight lifting
- I am eating and living healthy.
- I am drinking enough water to help me stay full and burn fat.
- I am now drinking myself to a balance weight
- I am eating more and more protein for muscle mass.
- I am eating less and less calories with every passing day.
- I am able to practice intermittent fasting
- I am eating more and more while foods.
- I am now a vegetable And fruit person
- I have drastically cut back on carbs.
- I have drastically cut back on sugars
- I am drinking more and more coffee for better metabolism.
- I have overcome the addiction for compulsive eating.
- I have overcome the love for refine carbs.
- I am health conscious.
- I am able to properly diet.
- I am able to slowly chew my food.
- I am eating more spicy foods for better metabolism.
- I am able to get better sleep
- Affirmations In Motion I allow myself to make healthy eating choices.
- My health is improving more and more every day.
- I am so happy and grateful now that I am reaching my ideal weight.
- My body is my temple and I lovingly take care of it.
- I choose to eat healthy foods that heal and nourish me.
- All the cells in my body are getting healthier every day.
- I easily resist all unhealthy food temptations.
- I enjoy life by staying fit and healthy.
- I always take care of my body.
- I love and accept myself.
- I forgive myself for all past weight loss failures.

- I now release all guilt I hold around past unhealthy lifestyle choices.
- I find it easy to reach and maintain my ideal weight.
- I love eating healthy foods that nourish my beautiful body.
- I visualize my ideal body daily and take action to make it happen.
- I choose to consume a nutritious diet.
- I am proud of myself for choosing a healthier lifestyle.
- Every cell in my body is becoming healthier and healthier.
- It is safe for me to lose weight.
- I have the power to change my life.
- I am surrounded by people who encourage and support me.
- I am confident of achieving my weight loss goals.
- I clearly see myself at my ideal weight.
- I am releasing any excess weight day by day.
- I love to exercise and move my body.
- I choose to eat foods that contribute to my health and vitality.
- I do what it takes to be healthy.
- It is fun and easy for me to lose weight.
- I easily obtain and maintain my ideal weight.
- I am capable of achieving my weight loss goals.
- I deserve to live a happy and healthy life.
- I am a weight loss success story.
- I am attaining my desired weight now!
- I am ready to accept perfect health and fitness.
- My body knows how to become balanced and healthy.
- I am becoming stronger and healthier every day.
- I love feeling empowered and confident.
- I allow my body to become slim and strong.
- Eating right and exercising gives me energy.

- I am getting slimmer and stronger every day.
- I find it easy to eat healthy.
- My metabolism is getting faster each day.
- I love feeling strong and slender.
- I am ready to let go of these extra pounds.
- I feel calm and confident about my body.
- I am letting go of fear and anxiety about my body.
- I give myself permission to be healthy and happy.
- I can achieve my weight loss goal with ease.
- I love and accept my body exactly as it is.
- I embrace the positive aspects of my body.
- I easily improve all aspects of my body.
- Loving my body makes sticking to healthy habits easier.
- My body loves being treated right.
- Cravings are just feelings; they will pass.
- I am strong enough to be slim and sexy.
- I can handle looking and feeling good.
- I am eager to embrace a slimmer me.
- I give myself permission to look and feel good.
- I choose to be balanced and healthy.
- I choose to take healthy actions for my body.
- I trust myself to make wise food choices.
- I am open to an abundance of well-being.
- I choose to think loving thoughts about my body.
- My body thrives when I treat it right.
- My health is improving every day.
- I am always aware of how certain actions affect my body.
- It"s okay to treat myself with love and kindness.
- My body processes food quickly and efficiently.
- Exercise energizes and strengthens me.
- I don"t have to be perfect, just try my best.
- I forgive myself for my poor eating and exercise habits.
- I am creating new, healthy habits one moment at a time.

- I am transforming myself from the inside, out.
- I deserve to be healthy, strong, and happy.
- I deserve to feel good about my body.
- I am proud of my commitment to treat my body kindly.
- I am willing to stick with this healthy lifestyle.
- I am committed to eating right and exercising every day.
- I crave foods that are good for me.
- My body thrives when I drink plenty of water.
- I trust my body to know what is best for it.
- I believe I can be slim, healthy, and beautiful.
- I approve of myself. You approve of yourself.
- I love myself. You love yourself.
- I support myself. You support yourself.
- I trust myself. You trust yourself.
- I am my best friend. You are your best friend.
- I become more lovable every day.
- My body is beautiful. Your body is beautiful.
- It is easy for me to forgive. It is easy for you to forgive.
- I forgive everyone. You forgive everyone.
- I forgive myself. You forgive yourself.
- I forgive the past. You forgive the past.
- I am free. You are free.
- I know life is for me. You know life is for you.
- I know what to do. You know what to do.
- I am capable. You are capable.
- I easily solve any problems. You easily solve any problems.
- I can handle anything that comes my way. You can handle anything
- that comes your way.
- I am full of praise and gratitude. You are full of praise and gratitude.
- I awaken each morning with joy. You awaken each morning with joy.

- I end each day with gratitude. You end each day with gratitude.
- I love my face and all my features.
- I am at peace with my body and form.
- I lovingly take care of my body.
- I love living in this exquisite female body.
- I adore my curves.
- I am sexy and attractive just as I am.
- I wear my confidence as well as I wear my makeup.
- I love my sleepy face and messy hair in the morning as much as I love it any other time.
- I appreciate the female cycles that my body experiences.
- I enjoy my body during sex and intimacy.
- I move my body with intention and love.
- I hold my head up high and wear a smile all the time.
- I love the woman I am just as Mother Nature intended me to be.
- I am the perfect height for me.
- I love the shape of my hands and the size of my feet.
- I wear my hair however it pleases me and I adore every strand.
- I like my thighs and my buttocks and take care of them with exercise and healthy eating.
- I am responsible for what I do with my body so I only do what's best.
- I choose to treat my body with care, love, kindness and respect.
- I push my body and marvel at the many ways it can bend, stretch, pose, move and breathe.
- I am enjoying a lifelong dance with my body.
- I am a strong woman.
- I look radiant by simply wearing a smile.
- I delight in taking care of my body when it needs healing and recovery.

- I channel love and energy to everyone around me.
- I listen to my body's needs with respect and kindness.
- I am patient with myself and worthy of all the waiting.
- I move at the perfect pace.
- I continue to be amazed by my body.
- I fill my body with confidence daily.

- I am confident
- Day by day my confidence is increasing
- Today and always, I am fearless
- Today I take action confidently
- Being confident comes naturally to me
- I am free of all fears of failure
- I am confident and determined
- I am naturally fearless
- I easily overcome any failures or setbacks
- I have one hundred percent trust in myself
- I am now bold and brave
- I am competent, smart and able.
- I believe in myself.
- My personality always shines forth
- I am outgoing
- I have overcome shyness
- I meet new people with ease
- I speak out with confidence
- I stay persistent and push through setbacks
- I can easily overcome any of life's hurdles
- I face anything that confronts me
- I am prepared for life
- Today I face my life head on
- I have full confidence in myself
- I have all the power I ever need
- I am in control of my life
- I easily tap into my own inner strength
- I go with the flow of life and succeed

- Being motivated and positive is normal for me
- I always succeed in spite of setbacks
- I am easy going, relaxed and social
- Confidence comes naturally to me
- I positive, friendly and confident
- I believe and love myself
- I stand up to anything
- I am naturally strong
- I was born with an inner strength
- I am confident
- My confidence is increasing
- I recognize the many good qualities I have
- I see the best in other people
- I surround myself with people who bring out the best in me
- I let go of negative thoughts and feelings about myself
- I love who I have become
- I am always growing and developing
- My opinions resonate with who I am
- I am congruent in everything I say and do
- I love and accept myself unconditionally
- I approve of myself and feel great about myself
- I radiate love and respect and in return I get love and respect
- I am a well loved and well respected person
- I am a cultured and wise and yet, a humble person
- My high self esteem enables me to respect others and beget respect in turn
- I am free to make my own choices and decisions
- I am a unique and a very special person and worthy of respect from others
- My high self esteem allows me to accept compliments easily and also freely compliment others

- I accept others as they are and they in turn accept me as I am
- It matters little what others say. What matters is how I react and what I believe
- All is well in my world and I trade love and acceptance with the world
- I have high self esteem as I respect myself
- I deserve all that is good. I release any need for misery and suffering
- I release the need to prove myself to anyone as I am my own self and I love it that way
- I am solution minded. Any problem that comes up in life is solvable
- I am never alone. The universe supports me and is with me at every step
- My mind is filled only with loving, healthy, positive and prosperous thoughts which ultimately are converted into my life experiences
- My mind is full of gratitude for my lovely and wonderful life
- I consciously release the past and live only in the present. That way I get to enjoy and experience life to the full
- Through confidence I can achieve anything
- I respect myself and I get respect from others
- I make every decision with total confidence
- I love and accept myself exactly as I am now
- I confidently face any challenge
- My confidence in my abilities increases every day
- I am becoming more confident every day
- I trust my inner voice to guide me
- I am well respected and well accepted person in the society
- I am the director of course of my life
- I am persistent and self reliant in whatever I decide to do

- I face challenges with courage and conviction
- I am proud to be me
- Friends love me and people respect me
- Myself belief grows daily
- My self esteem becomes better daily
- Self confidence is what I thrive on
- I enjoy life more with better self esteem
- I always go after what I want in life
- Confidence is my natural state of being
- Doors to amazing opportunities open to me
- Confidence is my second nature
- I am full of vitality and confidence

Affirmations to Condition the Body

- I have complete power over my health, wellness, and well-being.
- Daily in every way, I'm feeling more energetic and restored.
- I have the energy, vitality. and willpower to live a healthy whole life.
- I am healthy in every aspect of my being.
- I have complete power over my mind, body, and spirit.
- My energy vibrates radiant light, love, and power.
- My personal power is in complete harmony with my health, and wellness.
- I embrace my new vibrant body with joy, and gladness.
- I know my health is being completely restored back to its original state.
- I am calm, composed, and confident about my health.
- Every single moment that passes, I'm feeling better, stronger, and healthier.
- I am relaxed, centered, and refreshed in my present state of mind.
- I'm healthy, happy, and transformed.

- I give myself permission to heal.
- I'm filled with energy to do all my daily activities.
- I love and care for my body, and my body cares for me.
- My health is excellent, and I am perfectly fit.
- I have abundant energy, vitality, and a great sense of well-being.
- I know my life is in God's power of grace and restoration.
- I am now increasing all levels of energy – mentally, physically.
- I have control over my health and wellness.
- I use essential oils every day and in every way to support my health.
- I have abundant energy, vitality and well-being.
- I am healthy in all aspects of my life.
- I love my body and only feed it the best nutrition.
- I have no fear about being unhealthy because I know that I control my own body.
- I am always able to maintain my ideal weight.
- I am full of energy to do all the daily activities in my life.
- My mind is at peace and my heart is full of love.
- I love and care for my body and it cares for me.
- I'm healthy, happy, and transformed.
- I am unique and I love being ME!
- Essential oils work in perfect harmony with my body.
- I give my body permission to heal.
- I only eat what my body needs to be healthy and fit.
- I have released all my negative thoughts and replace them with positive ones.
- I have the stamina and energy to do all the things I love!
- I am now perfectly healthy in body, mind and spirit.
- I feed my body with proper nutrition.

- I am enjoying optimal health.
- I am mentally and physically fit.
- My health is excellent and I am full of life.
- I have abundant energy, vitality and well-being.
- I have a fit spirit, mind and body.
- I take 4 deep, relaxing breaths at least once each hour.
- I enjoy at least 8 glasses of fresh, clean drinking water.
- I do exercise and yoga upon arising every morning.
- I do 30 minutes of vigorous walking or aerobic exercise daily.
- I do strength training at least 3 times a week for my muscles.
- I am healthy, happy and radiant.
- I love to smile; it is my gift to the world.
- I am healthy and full of energy.
- I accept health as my natural state of being.
- I eat plenty of fresh fruit and vegetables to maintain my great health.
- Every day in every way, I am feeling energetic and enthusiastic.

Condition Your Mind Affirmations

- **Life loves me!**
- All is well in my world. Everything is working out for my highest good. Out of this situation only good will come. I am safe!
- It's only a thought, and a thought can be changed.
- The point of power is always in the present moment.
- Every thought we think is creating our future.
- I am in the process of positive change.
- I am comfortable looking in the mirror, saying, "I love you, I really love you."

- It is safe to look within.
- I forgive myself and set myself free.
- **As I say yes to life, life says yes to me.**
- I now go beyond other people's fears and limitations.
- I am Divinely guided and protected at all times.
- I claim my power and move beyond all limitations.
- I trust the process of life.
- I am deeply fulfilled by all that I do.
- We are all family, and the planet is our home.
- As I forgive myself, it becomes easier to forgive others.
- I am willing to let go.
- Deep at the center of my being is an infinite well of love.
- **I prosper wherever I turn.**
- I welcome miracles into my life.
- Whatever I need to know is revealed to me at exactly the right time.
- I am loved, and I am at peace.
- My happy thoughts help create my healthy body.
- Life supports me in every possible way.
- My day begins and ends with gratitude.
- I listen with love to my body's messages.
- The past is over.
- Only good can come to me.
- **I am beautiful, and everybody loves me.**
- Everyone I encounter today has my best interests at heart.
- I always work with and for wonderful people. I love my job.
- Filling my mind with pleasant thoughts is the quickest road to health.
- I am healthy, whole, and complete.
- I am at home in my body.

- I devote a portion of my time to helping others. It is good for my own health.
- I am greeted by love wherever I go.
- Wellness is the natural state of my body. I am in perfect health.
- I am pain free and totally in sync with life.
- **I am very thankful for all the love in my life. I find it everywhere.**
- I know that old, negative patterns no longer limit me. I let them go with ease.
- In the infinity of life where I am, all is perfect, whole, and complete.
- I trust my intuition. I am willing to listen to that still, small voice within.
- I am willing to ask for help when I need it.
- I forgive myself for not being perfect.
- I honor who I am.
- I attract only healthy relationships. I am always treated well.
- I do not have to prove myself to anyone.
- I come from the loving space of my heart, and I know that love opens all doors.
- **I am in harmony with nature.**
- I welcome new ideas.
- Today, no person, place, or thing can irritate or annoy me. I choose to be at peace.
- I am safe in the Universe and All Life loves and supports me.
- I experience love wherever I go.
- I am willing to change.
- I drink lots of water to cleanse my body and mind.
- I choose to see clearly with the eyes of love.

- I cross all bridges with joy and ease.
- I release all drama from my life.
- **Loving others is easy when I love and accept myself.**
- I balance my life between work, rest, and play.
- I return to the basics of life: forgiveness, courage, gratitude, love, and humor.
- I am in charge, I now take my own power back.
- My body appreciates how I take care of it.
- I spend time with positive, energetic people.
- The more peaceful I am inside, the more peace I have to share with others.
- Today is a sacred gift from Life.
- I have the courage to live my dreams.
- I release all negative thoughts of the past and all worries about the future.
- **I forgive everyone in my past for all perceived wrongs. I release them with love.**
- I only speak positively about those in my world. Negativity has no part in my life.
- We are all eternal spirit.
- I act as if I already have what I want—it's an excellent way to attract happiness in my life.
- I enjoy the foods that are best for my body.
- My life gets better all the time.
- It is safe for me to speak up for myself.
- I live in the paradise of my own creation.
- Perfect health is my Divine right, and I claim it now.
- I release all criticism.
- **I am on an ever-changing journey.**
- I am grateful for my healthy body. I love life.
- Love flows through my body, healing all dis-ease.

- My income is constantly increasing.
- My healing is already in process.
- There is always more to learn.
- I now live in limitless love, light, and joy.
- I become more lovable every day.
- It is now safe for me to release all of my childhood traumas and move into love.
- I deserve all that is good.
- **I am constantly discovering new ways to improve my health.**
- Love is all there is!
- My life gets more fabulous every day.
- Today I am at peace.
- Loving others is easy when I love and accept myself.
- I have the perfect living space.
- I have compassion for all.
- I trust the Universe to help me see the good in everything and in everyone.
- I love my family members just as they are. I do not try to change anyone.
- There is plenty for everyone, and we bless and prosper each other.
- I love and approve of myself.
- **Life is good, and so it is!**

Affirmations for Conditioning the Body

- Through these words I'm speaking now, I am physically and emotionally connected to an abundant source of healing.
- As I begin to focus more on how I can heal, new ideas and inspiration will come into my life.
- I welcome all perspectives, because anything can help me uncover new ways to feel better, live healthier, and love life more.
- I bow to the practice of being easy on myself. This reverence brings ease into my body.
- I'm willing to get as willing as possible to embrace the very parts of me that need love the most.
- Each day brings new priorities. I may want to focus on nourishing foods, or increasing my water intake, or taking a walk in nature, or choosing better-feeling thoughts. I embrace the message of each day and do my best to answer the calls from within, telling me what's best for this season of my life.
- I welcome all the people, things, events, and circumstances that will help me heal and grow.
- I have become a priority in my life. My health and healing matters. I'm worthy of a life that feels good to live.
- I am learning to be at peace with who I am now, and I'm excited about who I can be.
- Any insecurities I've been avoiding and perpetuating, may they be dissolved little by little each time I face them with a forgiving mindset and a self-compassionate stance.

- I'm ready to release the stories in my head and forgive myself for believing everything my inner critic has ever said. I know there is healing ahead.
- I'm actively learning to fall in love with taking care of myself.
- Every time I think healing thoughts, my body responds in kind.
- I choose thoughts that activate my potential for healing.
- I recognize any residual negativity in my mind and body, I hear its message, and I transform it into new, more helpful energy now.
- I have a healthy appetite for food that nourishes every cell in my body.
- I treat my body with respect because it's how I can best spread light on this planet.
- The non-physical in me honors the physical me.
- I'm ready to pay more attention to what I do like about myself and want for myself, instead of what I'm frustrated about not having or being.
- Self-compassion can help me respond to perceived setbacks in a healthy and hopeful way.
- I am dissolving old, painful patterns and letting a new pattern emerge.
- I know that everything isn't going to change all at once in a day, but I can make small choices in light of the larger picture.
- I can trade one moment of frustration for one moment of peace, one moment of self-defeat for one moment of self-compassion, and one moment of negativity for one moment of hope.
- I'm taking care of my thoughts when I'm alone and my words when I'm with others. I'm cleaning up my

life inside and out, and loving myself in the process; that's the only way to heal.
- I am deciding to get well. I am deciding to be well. There is no other option, no other alternative but for me to be well.
- Come what may, I can heal. This is a process to respect, but it's my clear and unequivocal decision, right here and now, to heal.
- If I'm not feeling well, I look to my most recent thought and choose the next available higher thought that makes me feel a little bit better. My mind is powerful.
- I'm not afraid to ask for help where I could use it. I'm not going to push myself further than my body is currently willing to go. I take each moment for what it is and follow the vision in my mind of where I'm going. I keep hope alive while honoring this step in the road.
- Well-being in all of its potential is all around me and within me, and I'm ready to receive it.
- I am grateful for the chance to be alive on earth, and I thank my body for allowing me this experience.
- I eat to fuel my body, not satisfy an appetite.
- Nothing tastes as good as being healthy and fit feels.
- What I do today shapes my today and creates my tomorrow.
- I will improve 1% each day and give myself pleasure for tiny progress.
- The past does not equal the future.
- This too shall pass.
- I love my life!
- All I need is within me now.

- Every day in every way, I'm getting better and better.
- Life doesn't happen to me, it happens FOR me.
- Everything happens for a reason and a purpose and it serves me.
- The best is yet to come.
- I am at peace with all that has happened, is happening, and will happen.
- Life is a gift and I enjoy each day fully.
- The more I focus my mind upon the good, the more good comes to me.
- The secret to living is giving.
- The smallest action can make a difference. My life is important. I can change the world just by being here, right now.
- Perfect health is my divine right, and I claim it now.
- I create my own beauty. I take care of my body, outside and in. I feel and look my best.
- I control how I feel – I can change my state in an instant.
- My home is a clean, warm, and happy place that supports my well-being.
- I am grateful for the riches in my life.
- I believe in my unlimited prosperity.
- I take massive action towards my goals everyday.
- I create money easily and effortlessly.
- My prosperous thoughts create my prosperous life.
- I honor my worth.
- I contribute and add value to the world everyday.
- Every cell of my body vibrates with energy and health.
- I am energetic.
- I am charismatic.

- Healthy food is a gift and a reward that I deserve everyday.
- My body is my temple.
- I make positive healthy choices.
- I have unstoppable energy everyday.
- I am a radiant being of light and spiritual love.
- I am always in harmony with the universe.
- I invite miracles into my life.
- I choose love, joy and freedom.
- I open my heart and allow wonderful things to flow to me.
- I love myself for who I am.
- I am a radiant person of positive energy.
- I am grateful for every moment of my life.
- I am comfortable with who I am.
- I am at peace.
- I attract only healthy, empowering relationships.
- I give and receive love effortlessly and easily.
- I have a fulfilling, loving and passionate relationship.
- My relationship is filled with love and passion.
- I am worthy of love.
- I am a source of love and inspiration for my family and friends.
- I am generous with love.
- I am blessed with a beautiful family.
- I am generous with my time.
- I am an amazing friend.
- Everything I touch is a success.
- I act promptly and decisively.
- I accomplish anything I put my mind to.
- I enjoy building my business everyday.

- My customers and visitors love the products and services I provide.
- If I am committed, there is always a way.
- My daily choices lead to my goals.
- My thoughts are positive and optimistic today.
- I learn from every experience in my life.
- Today is a winning day for me.
- I enjoy facing challenges that make me a better person.
- I feel great moving towards my goals today.
- My life is a series of successful choices.
- I live in the present and I live extremely well.
- Nothing keeps me from achieving my goals and living an amazing life!
- I can do all things through Christ who strengthens me.
- Abundance is God's will for me and I will not settle for less.
- The Holy Spirit is my helper; I'm never alone and I have the peace of God.
- I live by Faith, not by sight.
- At last, at last., the past is the past, I've broken free and won! Now is the time for me to have some fun!
- God's wealth circulates in my life. God's wealth flows to me in avalanches of abundance; all my needs, desires, and goals are met instantaneously by infinite intelligence; and I give thanks for all of my good now and for all of God's riches, for I am one with God and God is everything!
- I now command my subconscious mind to direct me in helping as many people as possible today to better htier lives, by giving me the strength, the emotion, the persuasion, the humor, the brevity, the confidence, the energy, whatever it takes to show these people and get these people to change their lives now!

- Now I am the voice.
  I will lead, not follow.
  I will believe, not doubt.
  I will create, not destroy.
  I am a force for good.
  I am a force for God.
  I am a leader.
  Defy the odds.
  Set a new standard.
  Step up
- Food is construction material for the body. I will become what I eat, as food literally becomes the cells, organs, and tissues of my body.
- Food is fuel. I will be as energetic as the fuel I put into my bodily engine.
- Nutritious foods contain everything I need for perfect health.
- When I feed myself nourishing food on a consistent meal schedule, it stokes my metabolic furnace.
- It's okay to eat for enjoyment or social reasons if I do it consciously and mindfully and I stay within the compliance rules and quantity limits I set for myself in advance.
- I'm totally conscious and aware of my beliefs about food and the reasons I eat.
- When I feel stressed or depressed, I have alternate ways to cope with those feelings.
- Healthy food that helps me burn fat and build muscle can be prepared in delicious ways.
- I realize that food can be one of life's great pleasures and that completely denying myself of foods I enjoy is not productive in the long run.

- I don't have to be perfect. If I eat healthy, natural foods at least 90 perfect of the time, I know I will get good results.
- If I set a compliance rule for myself, then there's no such thing as forbidden foods. As long as I obey the law of calorie balance and eat only small amounts, I can still be healthy, develop a great body, and enjoy my favorite foods in moderation.
- If I want better results, faster, I realize that I may need to tighten up my nutritional compliance and I'm willing to do it if that's what it takes.
- Everything I eat will have some effect on my body, but I realize that what I eat once in awhile doesn't impact me that much.
- What's most important is what I eat habitually, so I'm very conscious about what I eat repeatedly day after day. I understand and have great respect for the power of habits.

CONCLUSION

Lastly, if you enjoyed this audiobook I ask that you please take the time to review it on Audible.com. Your honest feedback would be greatly appreciated.

Thank you.

Now, I would like to share with you a free sneak peek to another one of my audiobooks that I think you will really enjoy. The audiobook is called "Positive Thinking: Be Happy and Love Life Powerful Subliminal Affirmations" Published by PMT Publishing.

It's an audiobook that provides you with affirmation that Condition Your Body and Mind to Natural Happiness. Program Your Brain to become Healthy, Attract Success and Abundance"

Enjoy!

Success Affirmation

I have the power to create all the success and prosperity I desire.

I let go of old, negative beliefs that have stood in the way of my success.

My mind is free of resistance and open to exciting new possibilities.

I am worthy of all the good life has to offer, and I deserve to be successful.

I believe in myself and my ability to succeed.

I am grateful for all my skills and talents that serve me so well.

I am enjoying my work today and optimistic about the coming days.

The universe is filled with endless opportunities for me and my career.

I am surrounded by positive, supportive people who believe in me.

I am always open minded and eager to explore new avenues to success.

Whatever I can dream up for my business, I can achieve.

I attract my ideal clients and customers with my energy. My ideal clients come to me easily.

I love every experience, client and prospect I've ever had.

My brand gives more value than it takes in financial gain.

My Business helps thousands and thousands of people. My brand solves real problems for real people.

My brand is always leaving people in a more positive state then when they began.

I have an authentic brand that creates and rallies people around a positive cause.

My brand is a leader in the industry. It paves the way for others to create and understand their reality.

My brand represents a set of positive values that I live my life by.

I am in business to help people, and to positively change the world.

I have an extremely engaged tribe and community that supports me.

My brand changes people, for the better.

I am passionate. I am outrageously enthusiastic and inspire others.

I allow my brand to be more than I've ever dreamed of. I am known for my positive energy and abundant lifestyle.

My positive attitude, confidence and hard work naturally draws in new opportunities.

I am enthusiastic and excited about my work.

My enthusiasm about my job is contagious.

My workplace is peaceful and full of love.

I make decisions easily.

I speak positively about my coworkers and they respond by speaking positively about me.

I am rewarded for doing my best.

I engage in healthy stimulation during my breaks.

I eat healthy, nutritious food during my lunch break and my body is grateful, granting me energy and good health in return.

I am an excellent employee, always productive and giving my best effort.

I am experiencing success in my career.

I enjoy working toward future career success.

I have a satisfying job.

I know exactly what I need to do to achieve success in my career.

My work environment is calm and productive.

The job I have is perfect for me.

I am experiencing wealth every day.

I am financially successful in all my endeavors.

I am getting wealthier each day.

I am living the life of my dreams.

I have enough wealth to fulfill my desires

I radiate success

I was born to be successful, it is my natural state of being.

The power is within me. I learn from the past, live in the now and plan for the future.

I am in control of my emotions, desires and abilities.

I trust in my capacity for greatness. I believe I am worthy of great success.

I live a beautiful life and I only attract the best of everything.

I am at peace with where I am and I have a strong vision for my future.

I am breaking through old, limiting patterns of behaviour and becoming more successful every day.

I love that opportunities to be successful are all around me, every day.

I celebrate the success I have in my life in every moment.

I am rich in love, wealth and happiness.

I recognize opportunity when it knocks and seize the moment.

Every day I discover interesting and exciting new paths to pursue.

When I need help, I effortlessly attract the perfect resources and solutions.

Everywhere I look, I see prosperity.

I am well organized and manage my time with expert efficiency.

I am committed to achieving success in every area of my life.

I love my job, and my work is a fulfilling part of my journey to greater success.

My ambitions are in perfect alignment with my personal values.

I work with fascinating, inspiring people who all share my enthusiasm.

By creating success for myself I am creating success and opportunities for others.

As I take on new challenges I feel calm, confident, and powerful.

Creating solutions comes naturally to me.

I always attract successful people who understand and encourage me.

I recognize every new challenge as a new opportunity.

I celebrate each goal I accomplish with joy and gratitude.

The more successful I become, the more confident I feel.

I consistently attract just the right circumstances at just the right time.

I am grateful for all the abundance flowing into my life.

I trust my intuition and am always guided to make wise decisions.

I stay focused on my vision and pursue my daily work with passion.

Every day is filled with new ideas that inspire and motivate me.

I excel in all that I do, and success comes easily to me.

I always expect a positive outcome and I naturally attract good results.

I take pride in my ability to make worthwhile contributions to the world.

I attract brilliant mentors who graciously share their wisdom and guidance.

I step outside my comfort zone with courage and confidence.

I am a patient listener and an effective communicator.

As I allow more abundance into my life, more doors open for me.

I am free of stress and I thrive under pressure.

I set high standards for myself and always live up to my expectations.

I have an endless supply of new ideas that help me become more and more successful.

I have released all limiting beliefs about my ability to succeed.

Every day I dress for success in body, mind, and spirit.

I think big and dream big without reservation.

I love who I am and I naturally attract people who respect me as a unique individual.

I am creating a life of abundance and happiness.

I am successfully living up to my full potential.

I am making the world a better place by being a positive, powerful influence.

I am grateful for my financial success.

I am living the dream!

My body is healthy; my mind is brilliant; my soul is tranquil.

I believe I can do anything.

Everything that is happening now is happening for my ultimate good.

I am the architect of my life; I built its foundation and choose its contents.

I forgive those who have harmed me in my past and peacefully detach from them.

My ability to conquer my challenges is limitless; my potential to succeed is infinite.

Today, I abandon my old habits and take up new positive ones.

I can achieve greatness.

Today, I am brimming with energy and overflowing with joy.

I love and accept myself for who I am.

Life supports me in every possible way.

I am in the process of making positive changes in all areas of my life.

It does not matter what other people say or do. What matters is how I choose to react and what I choose to believe about myself.

I am good enough.

I forgive everyone in my past for all the perceived wrongs. I release them with love.

I let go of all fear and doubt, and life becomes simple and easy for me.

Everything I need comes to me at the perfect time.

I feel glorious, dynamic energy. I am active and alive.

Today is going to be a really, really good day.

I am beautiful and everybody loves me.

I deserve only good in my life.

My good is constantly coming to me, so I relax and enjoy my life.

I can do it.

I deserve the best and I accept the best now."

I release all resistance to attracting money. I am worthy of a positive cash flow."

I practice forgiveness daily so that I cam free to move beyond the past into the present moment."

I love and appreciate myself."

"I act as if I already have what I want, it's an excellent way to attract happiness in my life."

"I am willing to change and grow."

I love every cell of my body."

I awaken today, appreciating everything in sight, and I give thanks.

I rejoice in the love I encounter every day."

All that I need to know at any given moment is revealed to me.

My intuition is always on my side.

I now free myself from destructive fears and doubts."

I am a unique and beautiful soul."

I am grateful for every experience I have ever had as it has shaped me into the person I am today, and that is exactly who I am supposed to be right this very moment."

I enjoy today and cheerfully look forward to tomorrow.

I choose to make the rest of my life the best of my life."

"I give my body what it needs.

I trust the process of life to always be here for me."

Today I mentally wrap each person I meet in a circle of love."

Abundance flows freely through me."

I am surrounded by love. All is well."

Life brings me only good experiences. I am open to new and wonderful changes."

I trust myself."

My mental pattern is positive and joyful."

I am a magnet for money. Prosperity of every kind is drawn to me."

Every moment presents a wonderful new opportunity to become more of who I am."

I lovingly do everything I can to assist my body in maintaining perfect health."

I am deeply fulfilled by all that I do."

I have plenty of time to do what I need to do.

Time expands for me."

I am an open channel for creative ideas.

I give myself permission to be prosperous."

I now see opportunities for abundance everywhere. I am blessed."

My day begins and ends with gratitude and joy."

I affirm that I have the power to heal myself."

Today I look at all the positive things in my life, and I am grateful for them."

"I have the knowledge to make smart decisions for myself."

I have all that I need to make today a great day."

I am, and always will be, enough."

"I acknowledge my own self-worth – my confidence is rising."

I let go of any negative feelings about myself or my life, and accept all that is good."

I always attract only the best of circumstances and I have the best positive people in my life."

I am courageous. I am willing to act and face my fears."

I have unlimited power."

I am a powerful creator. I create the life I want and enjoy it."

Every day I discover interesting and exciting new paths to pursue."

I trust my intuition and I always make wise decisions."

I am focused on my goals and feel passionate about my work."

I work well under pressure and always feel motivated."

I am living to my full potential."

I have everything I need to face any obstacles that come".

I have the power to create all the success and prosperity I desire."

I can let go of old, negative beliefs that have stood in the way of my success"

The universe is filled with endless opportunities for my career."

I am surrounded by supportive, positive people who believe in me and want to see my succeed"

I will be open-minded and always eager to explore new avenues to success."

As I take on new challenges I feel calm, confident, and powerful."

I will celebrate each goal I accomplish with gratitude and joy."

I choose to think positively and create a wonderful and successful life for myself."

Thank you for listening, this preview is now over.

I hope you enjoyed this preview of my audiobook "Positive Thinking: Be Happy and Love Life Powerful Subliminal Affirmations" Published by PMT Publishing.

Please make sure to check out the full audiobook on Audible.com

Thank you for listening.

www.ingramcontent.com/pod-product-compliance
Lightning Source LLC
Chambersburg PA
CBHW031151020426
42333CB00013B/604